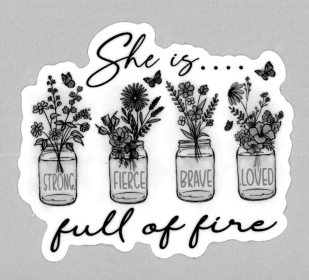

EARTH MEDICINES

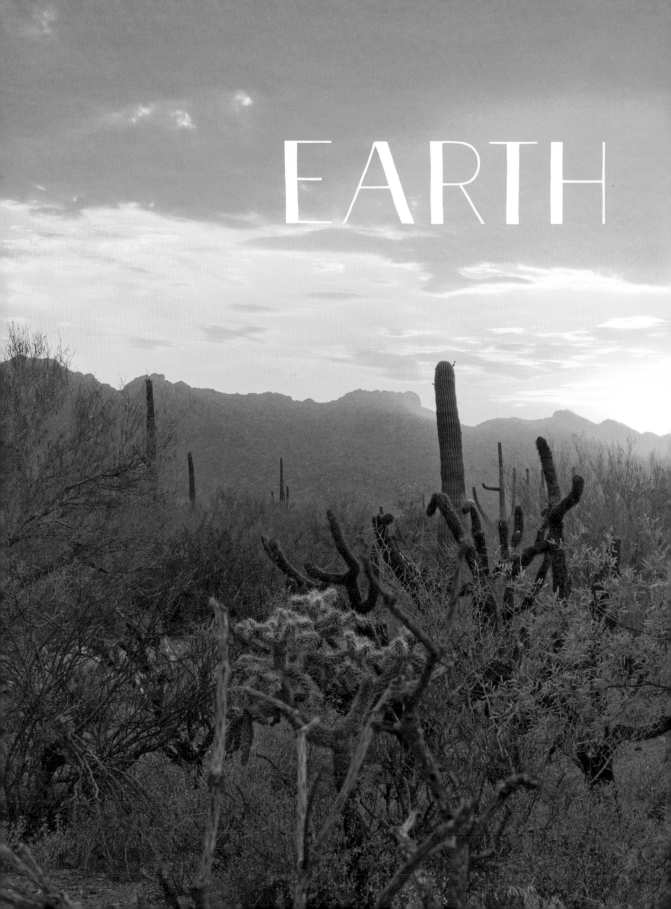

EARTH

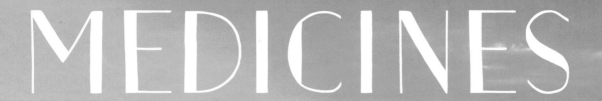

MEDICINES

Ancestral Wisdom, Healing Recipes, and
Wellness Rituals from a Curandera

FELICIA COCOTZIN RUIZ

PHOTOGRAPHS BY NICKY HEDAYATZADEH

RB

ROOST BOOKS

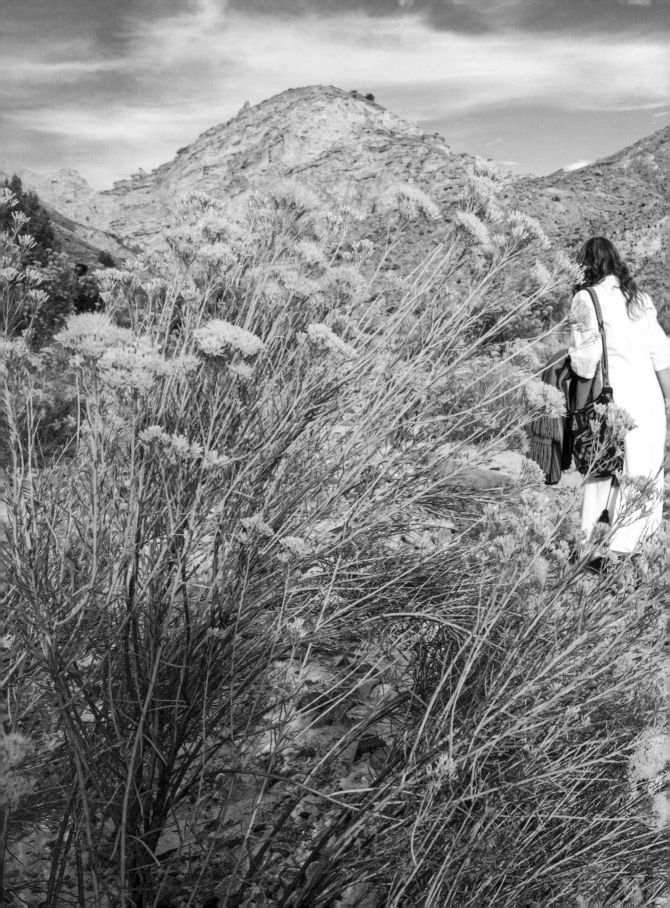

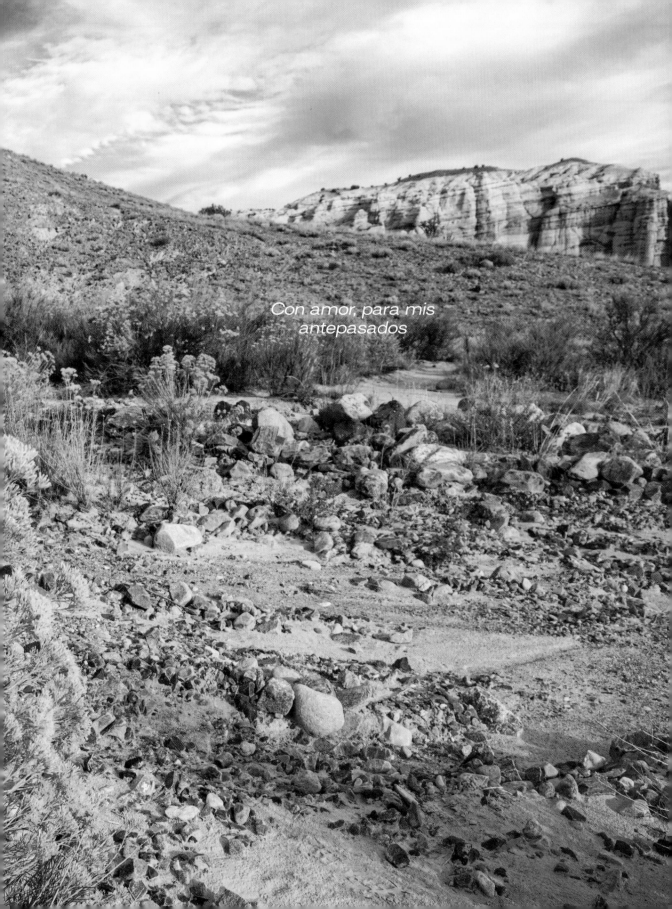

Con amor, para mis
antepasados

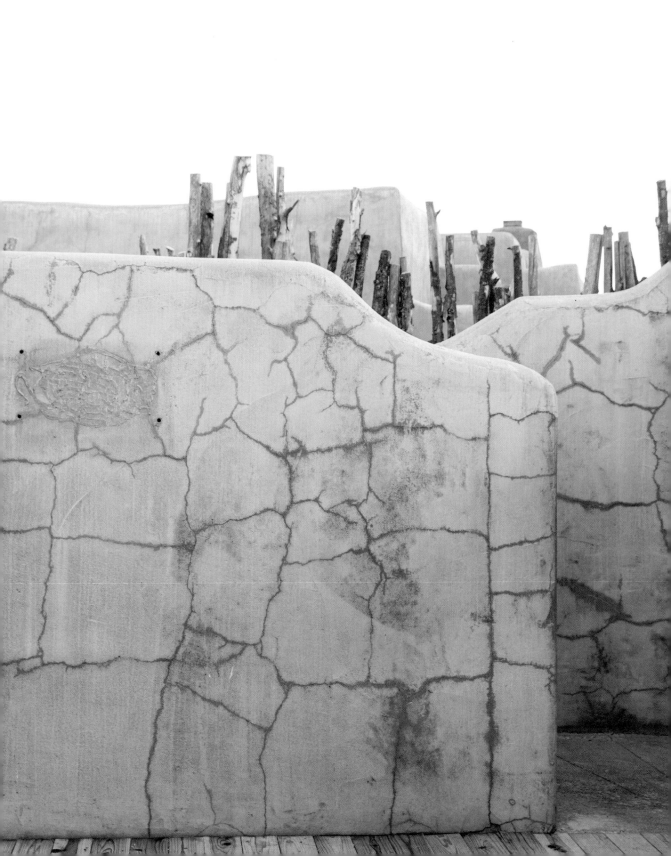

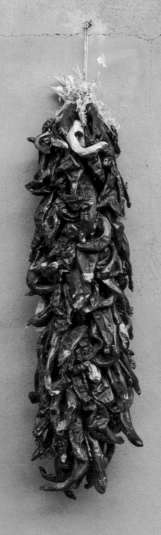

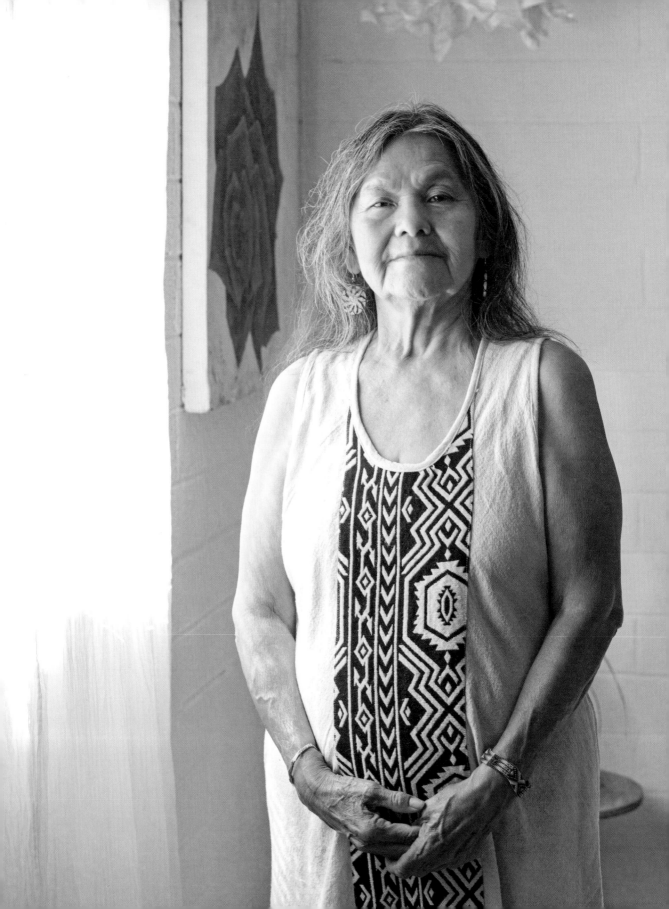

Foreword by Mona Polacca

I embrace you as beautiful relatives of the world, I offer you an open hand to show that I greet you in peace.

I am honored to share a few words about this wonderful book on behalf of my dear niece, Felicia Cocotzin Ruiz. She is from my father's paternal tribal family lineage of the Tewa Pueblo based in New Mexico, and we were filled with joy that after several generations, our paths in life connected through the parallels of our traditional Pueblo cultural upbringing!

Felicia has spent many years devoted to learning curanderismo and is well-known for her teaching about food as medicine throughout Indian Country and beyond. She reached out to me a couple years ago, telling me that she was beginning to develop her plan to write this book about how we, as Indigenous people, as well as others can use earth medicines—which Felicia describes as natural food, medicines, and healing based on traditional ways from all over the world—as a way to reclaim our health. She said, "I thought of you to write the foreword because of our meeting in Phoenix where you mapped out the Four Directions, explaining infancy, young adulthood, adulthood, and elderhood. My intention for this book is to share foods, remedies, and daily rituals with all readers, for the Circle of Life."

Writing this foreword is an opportunity to uphold my sacred relationship as a Koh-oh, aunt, in our Tewa way. My immediate thoughts on the topic were about how Indigenous people have historically eaten foods based on the seasons. These foods acclimated our body to the local seasons throughout the year. Thus, the seasons played a huge role in our health, as well as the ritual and ceremony of planting and harvesting food, and how we offer gratitude (reciprocity) before we enjoy eating it. Indeed, with the current pandemic and climate change, people are going back to the earth, interested in seeking knowledge on how to stay healthy in a holistic manner. So, this book is very important and timely for all of us.

I come from a culture that has been on the North American continent since time immemorial, surviving and thriving despite the many hardships and challenges. Over the ages, simple and fundamental truths have supported our survival, and I believe they are more relevant today than ever for society at large. Additionally, I believe that humanity needs to revisit its relationship with the natural world so that future generations of all people, plants, and animals may have a healthy future. Whether or not we think about them as spiritual or earth-medicine based practices, we all have an everyday existence that in some way incorporates the land we live on, the food we eat, the medicine we use, the language we speak, and the rituals we tend to. We share these practices with our family or tribal community. Yet, we hardly ever give much thought to how these practices are so crucially interconnected to our well-being—physical, spiritual, mental, and emotional. Yes, this book brings that all together as food for thought, and, of course, as food for nutritional health.

Did you know that many of the nutritious recipes for our meals today originate from Indigenous peoples? When you are informed about traditional knowledge, beliefs, and practices of the Indigenous peoples, what you eat and how you prepare your food could change your life for the better. I am sure that you have some family traditional recipes that have been passed down through the generations of your family. This is the same concept of passing Indigenous food and medicine knowledge. As Indigenous peoples, our teachings are relayed by word of mouth. Therefore, literature about our food- and medicine-ways from an Indigenous perspective is limited. Felicia's book offers teachings about how the positive aspect of both the foods you eat, and your wellness improves the quality of your own life.

Felicia has collected and created recipes and other bits of wisdom for over thirty years that can be applied by any kitchen healer to help remedy daily ailments for themselves or loved ones. She is giving you a peek into her notebook of remedies for all stages of life—from pregnancy to elder years—with the intention to give you a new way of thinking, a new approach to creative nutrition and wellness, and a new way of caring for your life. The recipes for food and self-care incorporate foraged and locally sourced ingredients, and Felicia also encourages you to explore the ingredients and medicines that can be found wherever you live. Along with recipes, Felicia's share her ideas for including ritual and ceremony in using these ingredients as medicine, both internally and externally. Besides the recipes, there are stories that will relate to and open up your own personal journey in life.

This book offers more than just recipes. It provides an opportunity for you to reflect upon your own personal relationship with food and medicine—how it is connected to identity and places of origin—and to remember the sacred nature of food, no matter who we are or where we come from. Food connects all of life and provides a pathway forward to reclaiming balance and peace with people and all of Nature. This potential exists through each ingredient's gift of nutrition, cleansing, and healing—both physically and spiritually.

I am very proud and in full support of the work my niece Felicia is doing to carry on the traditional wisdom and teachings that are a strong part of her ancestry. By stepping forward, between, and within cultures and languages, we can overcome boundaries. We can cross borders not only geographically, but also psychologically and spiritually. If we look at Earth from two hundred miles up in space, divisions do not exist, and it is very clear that we are one family on the Mother Earth. This simple point of view can guide us to act in a way that is life-sustaining, opening up a more inclusive worldview. We can listen more and have greater patience in finding solutions. So, I ask: Why not reframe or refresh your worldview and find the blessing within the recipes and stories Felicia shares with you? Allow for a moment of gratitude the next time you prepare and partake of the food or medicines you find in the pages of the book. Then, hope will flicker within—hope that allows us to envision a path toward a more compassionate and caring society that heeds the consciousness that Food is Life.

—**Grandmother Mona Polacca**, Havasupai/Hopi/Tewa, founding member of the International Council of Thirteen Indigenous Grandmothers and author of *Grandmothers Wisdom: Reverence for All Creation*

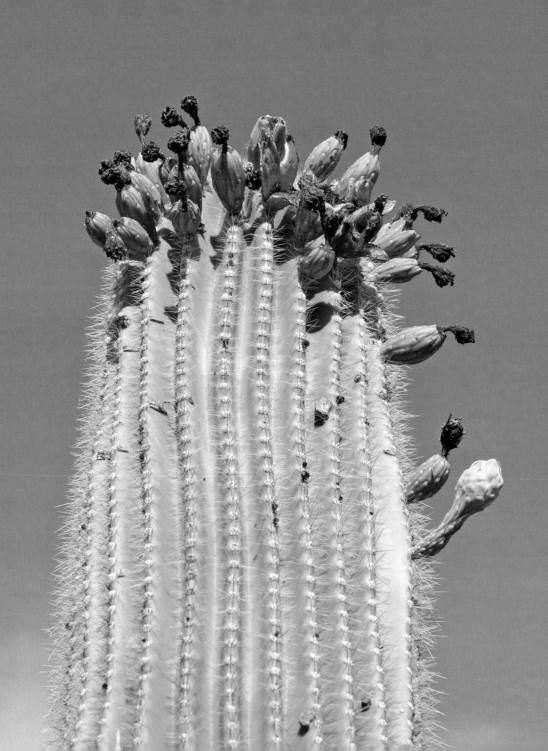

I live in the upper part of the Sonoran Desert, truly blessed to be among *all* of Earth's medicines. I was born and have lived in this part of the desert virtually my entire life, where days can easily reach 119 degrees in July and the rain has its own signature scent. This part of the world holds one of the most edible and medicinal landscapes of North America, and it is where some of my ancestors have cultivated their lives for thousands of years. This land, which includes mountain ranges, canyons, sand dunes, and even the sea, has helped raise me. It carries an energy like no other and speaks to me when I listen.

My cultural background extends far into Northern New Mexico, and I am Mexican, Spanish, and Tewa, all as a result of Spanish colonization. As a teen, I simply identified as Mexican, because that was the easiest answer to give to the common question "What are you?" which was usually followed by "When did your family get here?" When I felt like being more exact, I would proudly say I was "New Mexican," which was more confusing because that was often followed by the question "You're a 'new' Mexican?"

My Mexican ancestors, willingly and unwillingly, arrived in the late 1500s with the Spaniards, many as servants and laborers to settle in the northern territories of Mexico (now the state of New Mexico). Mixing with the Indigenous Pueblo People of the area and marrying or working for Spanish colonists caused large pieces of my Indigenous Mexican culture to be lost, while other important pieces survived including Nahuatl words, spiritual beliefs, and traditional healing ways. This is why the Southwest is so special to me. It *knows* how I feel. It has seen its own names and languages change, and it has witnessed firsthand the long history that my Indigenous ancestors carried on their backs and hauled in their carts—my culture and my roots. This is why I believe it has empathy for me.

Living *on* this land and later working *with* this land have allowed me to come full circle not only in my professional career but also as a person reclaiming their Indigenous roots. My work, which has changed over the course of my life, has always been rooted in traditional healing ways, beginning first with food.

Growing up Mexican in North Phoenix during the seventies meant my family was expected to assimilate to American culture, even though we were from "America." We lived and went to school in a predominately white neighborhood in which the principal and nurse encouraged my parents not to speak to us in Spanish, stating it would "not be good for our intelligence." Wanting the best for us, my parents followed their scholarly advice. Like many other Chicano kids of this time, our names were automatically Anglicized on our birth certificates by hospital staff, such as my brother's, from Andrés José (our grandfather's name) to Andrew Joseph. Like other kids, we ate peanut butter and jelly, except we made ours on flour tortillas.

My curiosity for cooking started at a relatively young age, in part because of my dad. Born in Northern New Mexico, he would share memories of his childhood that always intertwined food with other events. Memories of eating peaches from charred cans found in the rubble of a burned-down grocery store, drinking hot chocolate after nearly drowning in a flash flood, or quietly eavesdropping on his mother and her sisters while they laughed and told stories in the kitchen. His childhood memories sparked my imagination; I was always wondering what my grandma Lupita would cook for him since I never got to meet her. I now call this ancestral work.

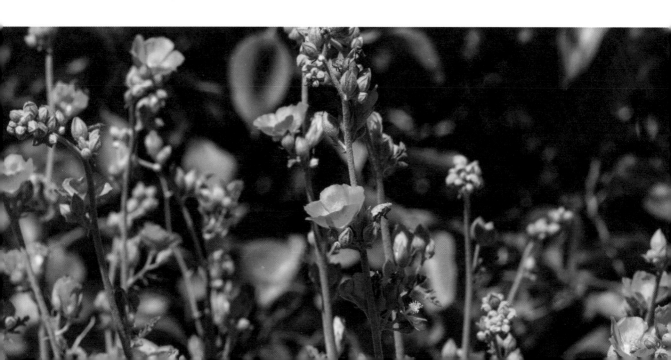

My passion for medicine making was sparked by another grand-mother, my Great-Grandma Delfinia, who had a relationship with plants, creating *remedios* for her community in Old Town Albuquerque. She was known affectionately as Grandma Chiquita because she was so tiny, and she is an integral part of my first memory of learning how to wildcraft plants. When we visited Grandma Chiquita during the summer months, we would take her to the mountains of her youth as well as visit my father's childhood village to reconnect to the land. It is there that I was introduced to plant medicine, following Grandma Chiquita with a paper bag as she gathered wild plants with her strong, wrinkled hands. Grandma Chiquita lived a hard life, helping to raise my mother under extremely poor conditions, yet she was always praying for everyone else's well-being. She lived to be ninety-four years old. It is through her life's example and from the stories I have heard about her that I learned about endurance and the power of prayer.

And then there was my brother Andy, whom everyone called a gentle giant. His death from HIV/AIDS in 1991 awakened me to the idea that I could use my hands as tools and work with life force energy. I was sitting at the end of his hospital bed, applying lotion to his size-fifteen feet when he said I should consider becoming a massage therapist because I had a good touch. I didn't think much about it at the time, but then I witnessed his spirit leave his body a few days later and saw how energy transformed right before my eyes. I realized my "good touch" was more about the cosmic energy shared between two people. It was that unsaid energy you feel when you enter a room or are near a person whose very being makes you feel a certain way. So, while massaging his feet and thinking comforting thoughts, I was unknowingly transferring good energy with my hands to his body. Two years later, I quit college and enrolled in massage school to start my formal training as a *curandera*.

In this book, you will see I often reference the traditional medicine of India called Ayurveda; I have studied various areas of this medical system throughout my learning including Ayurvedic massage, Ayurvedic cooking, and Yoga Nidra. Ayurveda has been practiced for thousands of years and works with the elements, herbs,

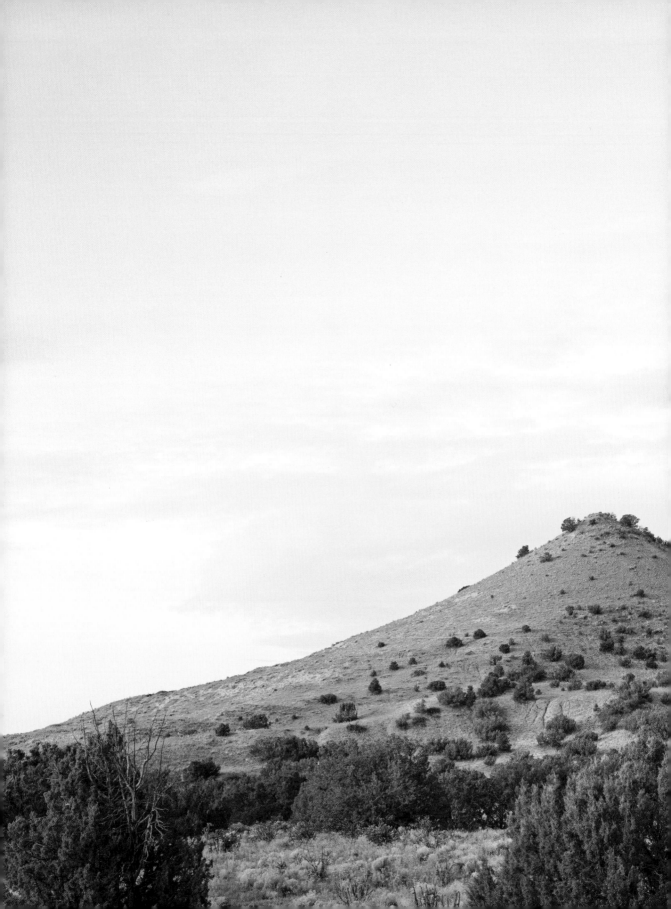

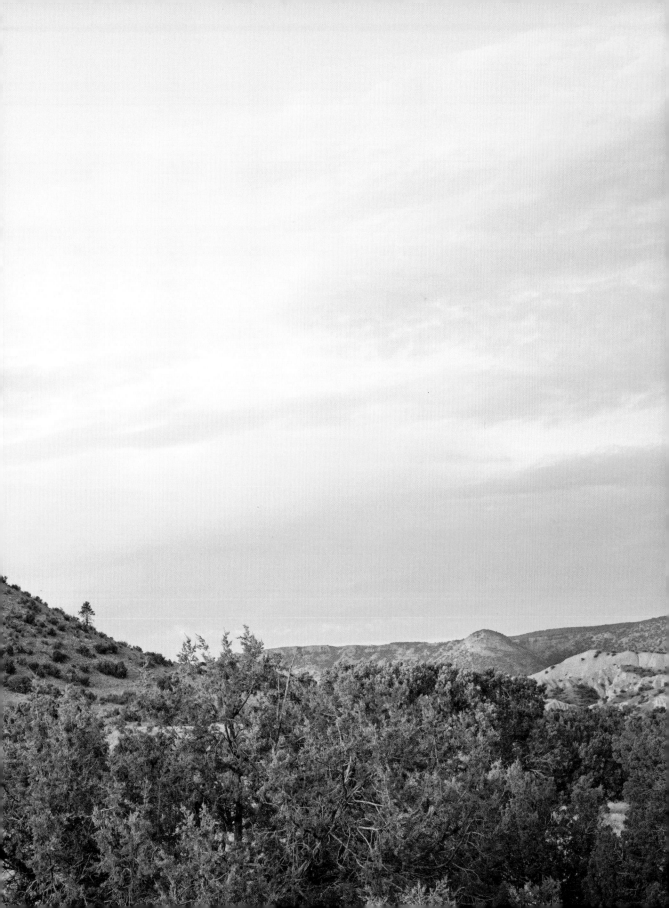

foods, and seasons much like *curanderismo*, which is why I believe I have a connection to this ancient practice. In Ayurveda, it is taught that energetic forces of nature manifest in our bodies as three different energies called doshas—*kapha*, *vata*, and *pitta*. And similar to curanderismo, it is believed that when these energetic forces are out of balance, they can affect our mental and physical well-being. To learn more about Ayurveda, I have included sources to learn from in the resources (page 203).

Massage school opened the door, but even before that, my life experiences were teaching my true being. Watching distant relatives dance in ceremony, wearing a safety pin of coral and turquoise as a talisman, walking with my great-grandmother to pick wild herbs on the hillside—those were cultural seeds that were planted in me in my youth, and I am harvesting them today. Yet, those memories and experiences also made me feel like I was from a space in-between.

I was confused about where our cultural ways fit in, as my formal learning clearly defined medicine by Eastern and Western traditions. Acupuncture, for example, is considered Eastern medicine, while allopathic care is considered Western. So, I wondered, if I am from here, what is *our* medicine? Is it East or West? Because although I live in "the West," our healing practices of working with energy and plants were closer to what was described as Eastern medicine. This in-between space led to a major shift in my thinking in my twenties. The two simple words, *Earth* and *medicine*, best described what my own healing practice was shaping to be: utilizing the elements, just like other Indigenous cultures found all over the world. I didn't want to use "East" and "West" when describing Earth medicines—it was a Eurocentric way of thinking, and also our traditional ways didn't seem to fit into those boxes.

This book is a culmination of that understanding. Weaving together a lifetime of working with natural medicine-ways has, in my own way, been an extension of *curanderismo*, whose foundation is a history lesson in itself. Curanderismo is a five-hundred-year-old traditional healing practice that is still in existence today. It is influenced by Spanish, Indigenous Mexican, West African, Moorish, and Native American medicine-ways as a result of the blending of those cultures during colonization. Curanderismo's use of the four elements—Water, Air, Earth, and Fire—is found deep in my culture. *Water* represents purity and transformation, serving as a foundation for many spiritual practices around the world. *Air* represents freedom, movement, and direction, and it works as a messenger, carrying the other elements. *Earth* is the collective home for all life, teaching us about cycles and reciprocity. And *Fire* is the transmutative energy that awakens our hearts and helps us move through times of great transformation.

Sprinkled with ancient spiritual insights from around the world, curanderismo is not a religion but rather a practice or understanding that the spiritual and the physical are interwoven and interact with one another. This "knowing" helped me understand more clearly the universality of other Earth medicines and spiritual practices, which is why I include stories and remedies shared by other cultures such as those of the Egyptians, who also worked closely with the elements. Like so many other traditional health systems connected to the Earth, curanderismo speaks to me personally as it reflects my Mexican lineage. This is why I encourage others to research their own cultural ways of healing in addition to trying my recipes and rituals. That way, you can uplift your own ancestors while fortifying your true spirit.

The recipes and rituals in this book are not meant to be—nor could they be—a manual on how to become a curandera or practitioner of traditional Mexican healing-ways. Rather, they are offered to share how acknowledging the elements playfully and more deeply, which is part of curanderismo, can help you keep harmony in your life. It took me twenty-three years to earn the title of curandera, and so it is important to me that I do not dilute the value of my own work, the journey of those on their curandera path, or the teachers who have helped me learn my traditional ways. This book is intended to help you build a closer relationship with the elements, using suggestions that have aided me and my clients and students. Many of the recipes and rituals are straightforward in how they include an individual element, while others are more abstract, connecting to the feeling of the element itself. You may resonate with some immediately, while others may require an open mind.

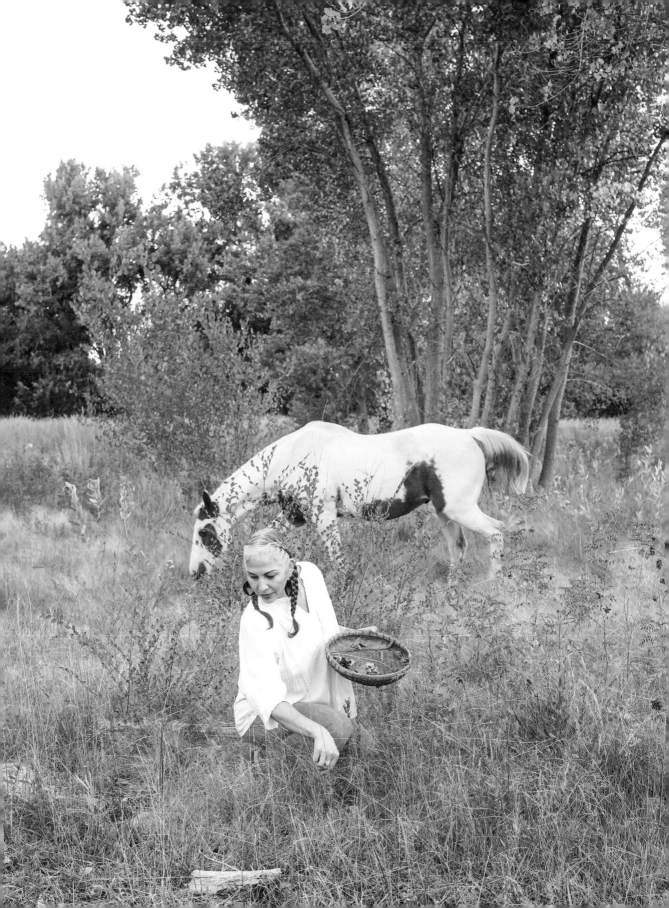

This book is divided into four parts, each recognizing and harnessing the power of one of the four elements. Within each part, I have organized the recipes and rituals so that when you are needing guidance, inspiration, or support working with the elements, you can look toward one of the three subsections. The first offers recipes for **inner harmony**, to nourish your body such as watering it with my Nopales Medicine Water (page 25). The second celebrates the **beauty** each element provides, such as nourishing your skin with my Corn Woman Facial Scrub (page 88). And the third integrates **spiritual work** to feed your spirit as with my La Guadalupana Cones (page 99) that use Mayan copal (tree resin) in an incense blend.

So, as with everything, I would like to start with an intention:

My intention for this book is to remind those who read it that we are all healers. Connecting with our Higher Source, our ancestors, and our inner lights, I pray all are divinely guided as they work with the medicines of Water, Air, Earth, and Fire. I pray that heart spaces open wide and feel the energy these medicines hold, and I hope gratitude is given daily to them for their gifts in helping us keep harmony of our beings.

Noxtin Nomecayotzin—To All My Relations,
Felicia

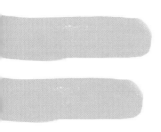

KITCHEN SUPPLIES FOR RECIPES AND RITUALS

When I think of what tools or supplies you may need to create the items in this book, I simply encourage you to be resourceful. I myself am extremely resourceful when making my own personal products, doing my best to use what I already have on hand. To me, this is part of living sustainably.

Many books I have read on cooking and herbalism often include lists of suggested tools and utensils, and this can make readers feel they have to go out and purchase all the items to do it "right." However, as exciting as it is to buy something new, there is much value in recycling and reusing. Many of my teachers were elders who were poor, and they created salves and herb bundles using empty jam jars, aluminum pots, coffee tins, and recycled flour sacks. Which is to say that it doesn't matter so much what you make or keep your medicines in. What matters is the medicines themselves! We live in a disposable culture, so shifting toward sustainable practices wherever you can truly does make a difference. Also, remember that when you throw something away, there is really no "away."

So, although the recipes in this book may include some supplies such as a 2-ounce glass bottle, if you only have a 1-ounce glass bottle, feel free to halve the recipe. Or, double it if you have a larger bottle. Think about saving and reusing what you may already have in your cabinet or refrigerator, and if you need something specific, hit your local thrift store or ask a friend. I often ask my close friends to save me small jars and bottles, and in exchange, I share my products with them. No one has ever said, "No thanks." That said, if you do need to order bottles or jars, buy them with the intention of reusing them.

Here are the tools I find useful for these recipes, but I urge you to be resourceful with what you already have.

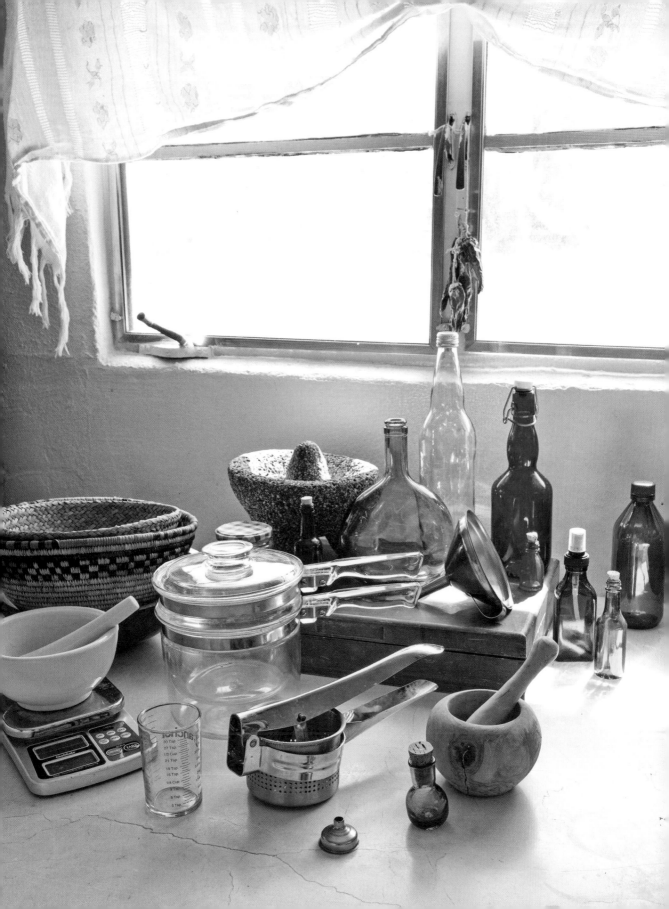

MORTAR AND PESTLE: This is a valuable tool—I have many. I use one for smashing garlic only so that my fragrant spices don't take on the flavor of garlic, and I also have my great-grandmother's *molcajete* (volcanic rock mortar and pestle) that I use only to grind dried chiles and spices.

POTATO RICER: This is a great old-school tool generally used to turn cooked potatoes into creamy mashed potatoes. I love using it to press out every single drop from an herb-infused oil instead of using an herbal press, which is better for large-scale production.

CHEESECLOTH AND NUT MILK BAGS: These are cotton pieces that, depending on their use, can be handwashed and reused several times. I use them often for my sun teas.

DOUBLE BOILER: Double boilers use steam as a heat source rather than the direct heat from the stovetop and are perfect for heating beeswax and solids such as raw cacao butter. If you do not have a double boiler, simply use a small pot or saucepan and a stainless steel bowl or Pyrex dish that fits over top. Add a few inches of water to the bottom pot and place it on the stove over medium heat with the bowl on top.

BOTTLES AND JARS: Jars and bottles of various sizes and shapes are ideal for many of the recipes in this book. Before reusing, give them a plunge in boiling water to sanitize them. Never use bottles or jars that held toxic chemicals for food or beauty products.

KITCHEN SCALE: This is a helpful tool for creating products so you can remember exactly how you did it later. Many of the recipes in this book are not exact, and experimentation is part of the process. Just a fraction of an ounce of beeswax can change the final result in a salve or balm, so always take notes when using your kitchen scale so you can make adjustments in the future.

BOWLS AND BASKETS: I was once told by a Diné elder that plants don't like to be in plastic. I do not know if the plants like nonplastic materials better, but I acknowledge the elder's advice. When I am collecting herbs or creating a blend, I turn to wooden, glass, or metal bowls for mixing and various baskets for drying and collecting.

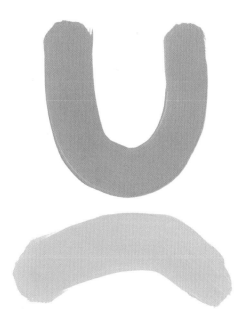

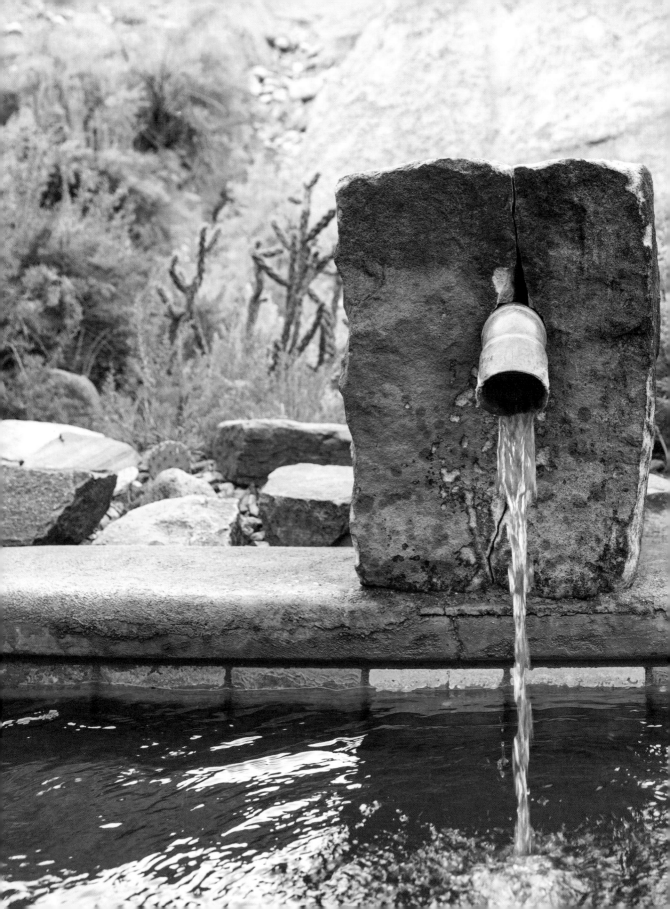

15 ◇ WATER

PRAYER TO WATER

Water, thank you for this gift of life. Thank
you for reminding me to go with the flow
and to allow events in my life to unfold
naturally. Your properties remind me to
be adaptable and to honor my personal
boundaries. Flow through my body and
return to the Earth as medicine. May rivers
of compassion stream from my heart for
those who live without access to your
sweet waters.

WATER FOR INNER HARMONY

THE BEAUTY OF WATER

SPIRITUAL WORK WITH WATER

WATER IS A MAGICAL SHAPESHIFTER

It can physically change from solid to liquid to gas. It can be steam, bursting deep from within the Earth, or a delicate six-sided snowflake, falling from the sky. Water is receptive; it holds, carries, and pours. Water listens. We, as humans, have always had a close and crucial relationship with Water. It has been scientifically shown to respond to positive and negative words, just as we humans do. Mother Earth is covered with 71 percent Water and our own bodies are 78 percent Water at birth. In the womb, Water was our first home, therefore our first medicine. Everything is connected to Water.

In my own culture, we have many associations with Water, one being Chalchiuhtlicue, the Mexican Water goddess. She represents the purity and preciousness of Water through fresh springs, peaceful rivers, and birthing rituals; however, she is also feared because she has the power to drown people and overturn boats. Like Water itself, she is transformative and ever-changing.

Water also represents new beginnings. In Southern Arizona, I learned how to harvest fruit from the saguaro cactus with one of my plant teachers named Teresa, a Tohono O'odham elder. Teresa taught me that the Tohono O'odham New Year celebration begins with the changing of spring to summer, signaled by the powerful monsoon rains bringing life-giving Water. So, it was extra special collecting these delicious fruits, knowing we were also celebrating the new year together at each summer harvest.

As we are fundamentally made of Water, working with this element helps people return to their physical Self. Staying well-hydrated can help you feel more energetic, achieve a dewy complexion, and aid in detoxing impurities from your body. The body uses Water internally for virtually every function, including carrying oxygen, moistening tissues, and transporting hormones. Water is also crucial in maintaining optimal cellular functioning and the support of the aging process. Some of the best ways to keep skin hydrated are with humectants, substances that *draw* Water from the Air to the skin such as aloe vera gel, and occlusives, substances that form a protective layer to *seal* Water in such as beeswax and shea butter.

Water's natural abilities to soften and dissolve support us when we need to wash away fears and negative emotions. There is no life without Water, which is why it is the foundation for so many spiritual practices in various cultures around the world—from the River Ganges in India to the sacred cenotes of the Yucatán Peninsula. Creation stories and Water deities that symbolize rain and the giver of life have been passed down orally and are still shared today among many Indigenous cultures. At one point in time, every culture on Earth considered Water to have great spiritual value, using it in ceremony, initiations, and cleansings. Though many cultures still recognize these spiritual uses, sadly, careful consideration and reverence for this precious element are not widespread anymore. In the following sections, you will find small ways you can reconnect to the energies of Water, learning how to listen to it and work with it once again.

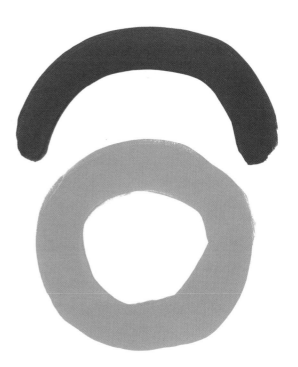

WATER
FOR INNER
HARMONY

HYDRATING SKIN FOOD

Eating fresh foods that have naturally high water content such as melon and celery hydrates your body from the inside out. These foods are also often high in vitamin C, which supports and maintains collagen production. When my daughter was a preteen, I called them "skin foods," which was a great strategy to get her interested in healing foods at an age when many struggle with skin issues such as acne or eczema. Here are some easy and delicious recipes, filled with her favorite skin foods.

RADIANCE BOOSTING CUCUMBER SALAD

Serves 2

Cucumbers are over 95 percent water, making them one of the most hydrating foods for our bodies. Fresno chiles, like all chiles, are high in vitamin C, while ginger contains powerful anti-inflammatory properties called gingerols that can help soothe irritated skin.

> 1 English cucumber, unpeeled, washed and trimmed
> 1 Fresno chile, seeded, minced
> 1 teaspoon fresh ginger, unpeeled, grated
> 2 tablespoons raw apple cider vinegar
> 2 tablespoons tamari
> Agave syrup
> 1 tablespoon black sesame seeds

Thinly slice the cucumbers width-wise into rounds with a sharp knife or mandoline and arrange them on a platter or in a bowl. In another small bowl, mix together the chile, ginger, apple cider vinegar, tamari, and a drizzle of agave syrup. Using a spoon, dress the cucumber slices with the dressing and garnish them with black sesame seeds.

(continued)

BRIGHT AVOCADO AND WATERMELON RADISH PLATTER

Serves 2

The water content of avocados averages 75 percent, and they are bursting with nutrients such as vitamins A and E. Watermelon radishes are nearly 90 percent water and are an absolutely beautiful bright-pink color when you slice them open. That color is where the name comes from, as they don't taste like watermelon! They are actually part of the mustard family and have a crisp, peppery flavor.

2 cups arugula
1 small watermelon radish, thinly sliced
1 large avocado, peeled and sliced
1 tablespoon olive oil
½ large lemon, juiced
Sea salt
Ground black pepper

Arrange the arugula on a plate or platter in one layer. Arrange the radish slices over the arugula in one layer. Arrange the avocado slices over the radish in one layer. Drizzle the salad with olive oil and lemon juice, and season with salt and pepper.

(continued)

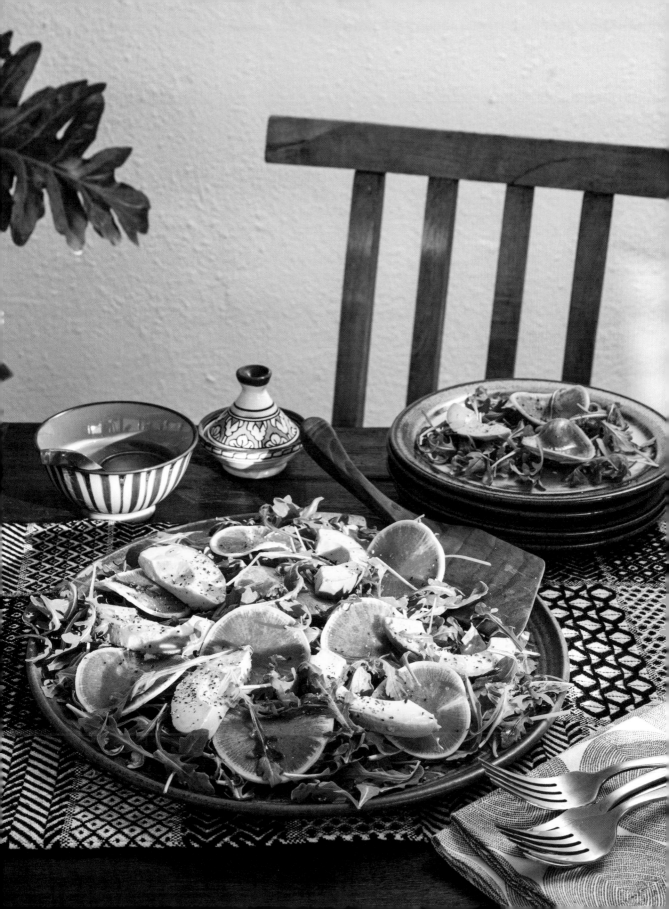

SWEET ANISE CITRUS SALAD
Serves 2

Sweet anise, also called fennel, is one of my favorite herbs, flavor-wise. Pairing its licorice–like flavor with tart citrus is a popular combination. Both are packed with vitamin C, helping with skin texture and moisture. When purchasing sweet anise, look for bulbs that come with their fronds so you can use them as garnish.

1 large grapefruit or 2 medium oranges

½ small sweet anise bulb, thinly sliced; fronds minced, if available

¼ cup Marcona almonds

Olive oil, for drizzling

Sea salt

Ground black pepper

Begin by slicing the top and bottom off each citrus fruit to reveal the flesh. Set one of the cut sides down on the cutting board and use your knife to trim off the peel and as much white pith as possible. Once peeled, turn the citrus on its side and slice into ½ inch rounds. Then, arrange the citrus and sweet anise on a platter. Sprinkle the salad with almonds, add a drizzle of olive oil, and season with sea salt and pepper. Garnish with the minced fronds.

AGUAS FRESCAS

Aguas frescas translates as "fresh waters" in Spanish and are refreshing drinks found year-round in Mexico City street carts. They are typically made with seasonal fruits and water and are sweetened with sugar. Although they are super refreshing on a hot day, I find many of them overly sweet for my own liking.

This inspired me to create *aguas medicinales* (medicine waters) by reducing or omitting the sugar and including cooling herbs, chia seeds, and more. The result is a healing water that delivers moisture and restorative vitamins to the body.

NOPALES MEDICINE WATER

Makes 4 servings

4 cups water

1 cup fresh nopales, de-spined, rinsed, chopped (see note)

1 cup fresh basil

2 large limes, juiced

1-inch piece fresh ginger, peeled

Natural sweetener (honey or maple syrup, optional)

Nopales are cactus pads from the nopal cactus. They are readily available cleaned and de-spined in most Mexican or Latino grocers.

Put the water, nopales, basil, lime juice, and ginger in a blender and pulse until smooth, adding more water if needed to achieve the desired consistency. Add a sweetener of your choice to taste. Serve chilled or over ice.

(continued)

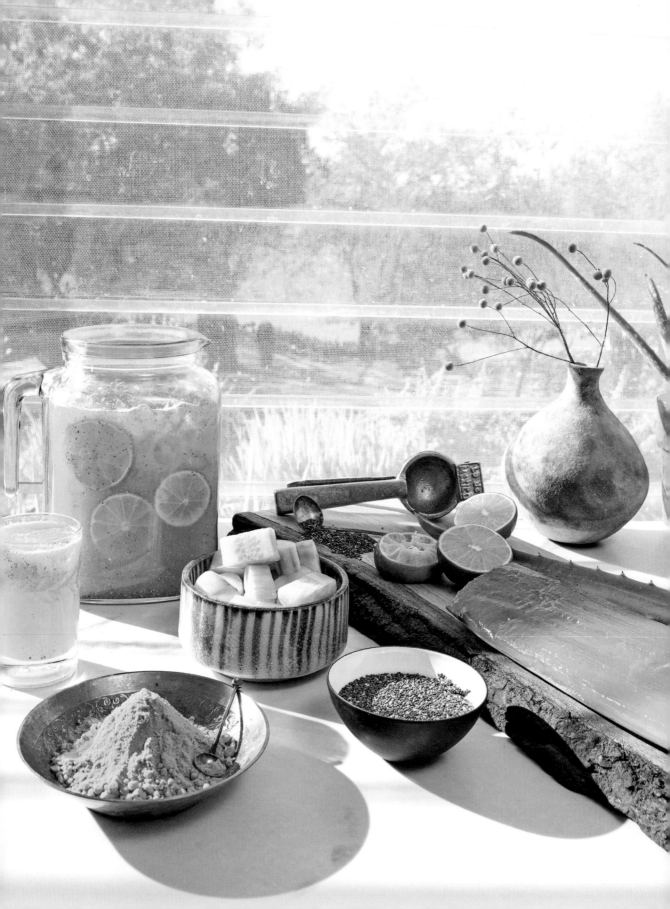

CUCUMBER ALOE VERA MEDICINE WATER

Makes 4 servings

4 cups water

1 large cucumber, peeled, chopped

1 cup fresh lime juice

1 teaspoon ground turmeric

1 tablespoon chia seeds

½ cup fresh aloe vera gel, store-bought for consumption
or harvested from an aloe vera leaf (see below)

Natural sweetener (honey or maple syrup, optional)

Put the water, cucumber, lime juice, turmeric, chia seeds, and aloe gel in a blender (working in batches if necessary) and pulse until smooth, adding more water if needed to achieve desired consistency. Add a sweetener of your choice to taste. Serve chilled or over ice.

How to Prepare Aloe Vera Gel

You can find fresh aloe vera leaves at most Mexican grocery stores. To prepare the aloe vera gel, first trim the base and the top of the leaf. Drain the aloin (yellow substance) from the leaf by placing it in an upright container or in your kitchen sink for about 10 minutes. You will see the aloin ooze out from the bottom. Although it is not toxic, it has a strong bitter flavor. After 10 minutes, place the aloe vera with the flat side down on a cutting board and slice off the spiny sides. Using a vegetable peeler or small paring knife, remove the bright-green layer. Use a spoon to remove the gel or slide your knife under the gel to carefully release it from the other side. You can now cut your gel into small pieces and refrigerate.

AYURVEDIC COPPER WATER

In the ancient practice of Ayurveda, drinking copper-charged water in the morning is recommended for maintaining good health. Called *tamra jal*, it is made by storing water overnight in a copper vessel and is believed to help balance all three *doshas* in the Ayurvedic system of healing. When water is stored in a copper vessel for at least 8 hours, a very small amount of copper ions gets dissolved into the water, resulting in positively charged water.

Copper is packed with antioxidants and cell-forming properties that fight off free radicals, which makes it helpful in the production of new and healthy skin cells. Copper also has anti-inflammatory properties that can help with arthritis and other inflammatory pains. Making your own Ayurvedic copper water is simple and something I include in my morning ritual.

Copper oxidizes naturally and needs to be cleaned every few months. Traditional Indian methods of cleaning copper include rubbing the copper with a mixture of salt and either tamarind paste or fresh lemon juice. To clean my copper pitcher, I cut a lemon in half, dip one half in sea salt, and scrub the outside of the pitcher with the salted lemon. It brightens up nicely.

Pure copper vessel
Water

Fill your copper vessel with water in the evening and leave it in the vessel overnight or for at least 8 hours. In the morning, enjoy a cup of energized copper water.

GREEN WATER WELLNESS SHOTS

Tecuítlatl, known more commonly as spirulina, is one of my Mexican ancestral foods. It is a type of blue-green algae, of which there are many edible species. Blue-green algae are found on all continents (except Antarctica). Tecuítlatl roughly translates as "secretions of the stones" in Nahuatl, and it is one of the oldest and most nutrient-dense foods on Earth. Sixteenth-century Spanish chroniclers noted that spirulina was traditionally collected from the surface of alkaline lakes in the Mexican basin, where it was then dried into little cakes to be rehydrated or consumed in its powdered form. Unfortunately, the Mexican lakes producing spirulina were drained as part of the Spanish conquest, and the blue-green algae were forgotten for many generations. I am so grateful this richly pigmented food source has made a comeback and is now easily found in many stores.

The benefits of spirulina include exceptionally high levels of vitamins, minerals, and micronutrients. Aside from being a great immune supporter, it also has essential fatty acids, which help your skin's cells retain moisture.

Makes 2 servings

1 large lemon, juiced (about ¼ cup)

1 teaspoon powdered spirulina

1 teaspoon natural sweetener (honey or maple syrup)

Place all the ingredients in a small jar, cover, and shake well. Pour the drink into two shot glasses and enjoy first thing in the morning or when you need a little pick-me-up.

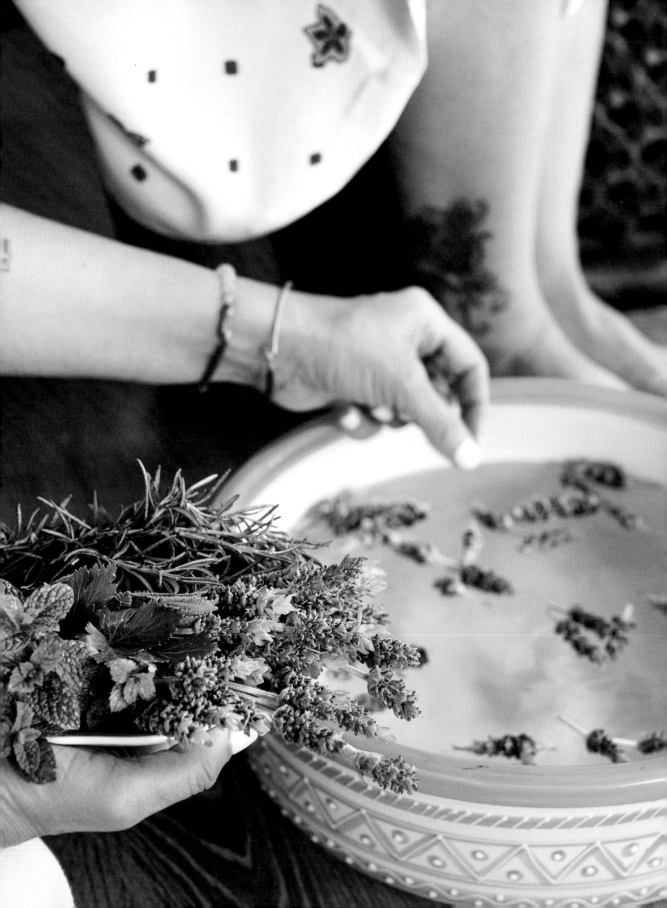

HYDROTHERAPY FOR HEADACHE RELIEF

I suffered from regular migraines, beginning as a teenager and well into my thirties. And although I have learned what most of my triggers are, every now and then, I am still plagued with a debilitating headache. My migraines typically last from half a day to a full day, with the classic symptoms of nausea, throbbing pain, and light sensitivity. One remedy I find most helpful during a migraine is hydrotherapy. Hydrotherapy uses hot and cold water to improve the circulation of the blood and lymph in the body.

Migraines are a source of discomfort because they cause the blood vessels in your head to get bigger, therefore circulating too much blood to your head. In hydrotherapy, cold water applied to the head and neck constricts the blood vessels. Simultaneously, hot water applied to the feet does the opposite. With the blood vessels near the head becoming smaller and those in the feet becoming bigger, blood begins to circulate down to your feet. Essentially, the cold water pushes the blood away from your head and the warm water welcomes it down to your feet.

I learned about this treatment firsthand from my old roommate and dear friend, the herbalist Aztechan Pettus. At the time, she was also an aromatherapy instructor. Her gentle touch and confidence in knowing exactly what to do in the moment relieved my pain quickly. I was so lucky we were roommates, and she has continued to share her knowledge with me and so many others over the years.

This therapy is simple to put together if your pain threshold is low enough to do so; if not, ask a friend or family member to assist if possible.

(continued)

Makes one treatment

**A handful of one, or a combination of the following: fresh
ginger slices, fresh lavender, fresh mint, or fresh rosemary**
Medium bowl
Small towel
Large bowl
Bath towel

Fill the medium bowl with ice water. Soak the small towel into the
ice water, wring it out, and place it on your forehead or the back of
your neck. Put the large bowl filled with warm water on the floor
and have the dry bath towel nearby. Place your feet into the warm
water. Add the fresh herbs. Sit comfortably with your eyes closed in
a quiet space for 15 to 20 minutes, out of direct light. Take caution
to not slip when stepping out of the water by using the bath towel
to dry your feet. Rest afterward.

Water Therapy

My husband, Jason, is a physical therapist who is trained in a type of water therapy
called Watsu. Developed at Harbin Hot Springs in California, the modality's creator,
Harold Dull, found that warm water was the ideal medium to practice Zen Shiatsu
massage, hence the name Watsu. My husband finds this therapy very effective
for his patients who are living with brain and spinal cord injuries. It relieves muscle
tension and chronic pain while creating an overall feeling of centeredness. The work
is very intimate, with the patient and practitioner submerged in chest-high water
that is heated to 94 to 98 degrees. This temperature is thought to create a state of
homeostasis, which allows the body to completely relax. The practitioner supports
the head of the patient with one arm and employs his other arm to support their
back, cradling the body as it moves gently in the water.

There are many forms of water therapy, some incorporating flotation devices and
breathwork, but it is the water itself that is the most important tool; it removes the
effects of gravity by taking the weight off the joints thus creating more freedom and
movement. Although each therapy may vary in technique, they all utilize a form of
stretching movements to promote relaxation of the muscles while offering a deep
sense of well-being. It truly is a body and mind experience.

Many local spas, wellness resorts, and gyms offer water therapy with many
practitioners also offering in-home sessions.

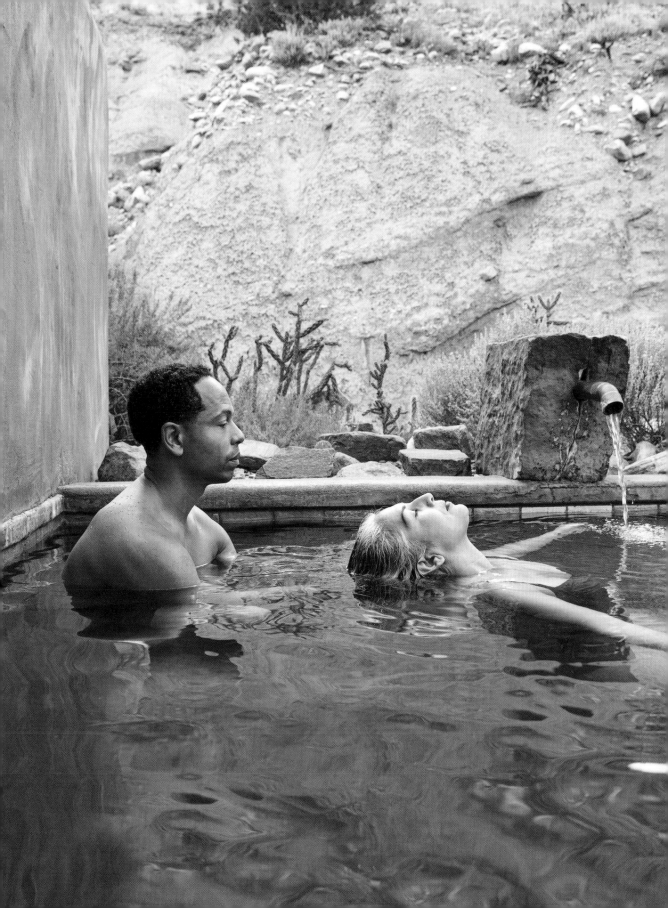

THE
BEAUTY
OF WATER

BOTANICAL HYDRATING MISTS

Facial mists made from dried herbs are one of my personal feel-good beauty products. They are physically hydrating to the skin and impart a delicate scent perfect for your morning ritual. You can use distilled water, reverse osmosis water, or even pure rainwater if you live in an area where collecting fresh rain is a possibility. The important thing is to use water that is free of contaminants. Below are recipes you can personalize for your own skin type.

SOOTHING CALENDULA MIST FOR SENSITIVE SKIN

Makes about 1 cup

¼ cup dried calendula flowers

1 cup water

1 tablespoon aloe vera gel (see page 27)

1 drop chamomile essential oil

Optional:

Dry Skin: Add 1 teaspoon avocado oil or 1 teaspoon jojoba oil

Oily Skin: Add 1 teaspoon organic witch hazel extract

8-ounce dark glass bottle with mister

Place your calendula flowers and water in a small saucepan and bring the mixture to a boil. Reduce the heat and simmer for 5 minutes. Remove the pan from heat and allow the mixture to cool to room temperature. Using a fine mesh strainer, strain the flowers over a glass measuring cup, pressing the mixture with the back of a spoon to extract as much liquid as possible. You can also use a potato ricer to squeeze out every last drop. Add the aloe vera gel, essential oil, and your dry skin or oily skin ingredient (if using),

(continued)

and mix with a spoon. Using a funnel, fill the glass bottle with the botanical water, storing any remainder in a tightly capped jar or bottle in the refrigerator. To use, lightly spray the face to hydrate and refresh your skin.

MORNING RITUAL GENTLE MIST

Makes about 1 cup

½ cup dried lavender

½ cup dried rose petals

1 cup water

Optional:

Dry Skin: Add 1 teaspoon avocado oil or 1 teaspoon jojoba oil

Oily Skin: Add 1 teaspoon organic witch hazel extract

8-ounce dark glass bottle with mister

Place your dried flowers and water in a small saucepan and bring the mixture to a boil. Reduce heat and simmer for 5 minutes. Remove the pan from heat and allow the mixture cool to room temperature. Using a fine mesh strainer, strain the flowers over a glass measuring cup, pressing the mixture with the back of a spoon to extract as much liquid as possible. You can also use a potato ricer to squeeze out every last drop. To the measuring cup, add your dry skin or oily skin ingredient (if using), and mix with a spoon. Using a funnel, fill the mister bottle with the botanical water. If you are using a smaller bottle, store the remainder in a tightly capped jar or bottle in the refrigerator. To use, lightly spray your face to hydrate and refresh your skin.

VITAMIN C BOOSTER FOR DULL SKIN

Makes about 1 cup

½ cup dried hibiscus flowers

½ cup dried rose hips

1 cup water

Optional:

    Dry Skin: Add 1 teaspoon avocado oil or
1 teaspoon jojoba oil

    Oily Skin: Add 1 teaspoon organic witch hazel extract

8-ounce dark glass bottle with mister

Place dried herbs and water in a small saucepan and bring mixture to a boil. Reduce heat and simmer for 5 minutes. Remove the pan from heat and allow mixture to cool to room temperature. Using a fine mesh strainer, strain the hibiscus flowers and rose hips over a glass measuring cup, pressing the mixture with the back of a spoon to extract as much liquid as possible. You can also use a potato ricer for the same result. To the measuring cup, add your dry skin or oily skin ingredient (if using), and mix with a spoon. Using a funnel, fill the mister bottle with the botanical water. If you are using a smaller bottle, store the remainder in a tightly capped jar or bottle in the refrigerator. To use, lightly spray your face to hydrate and refresh your skin.

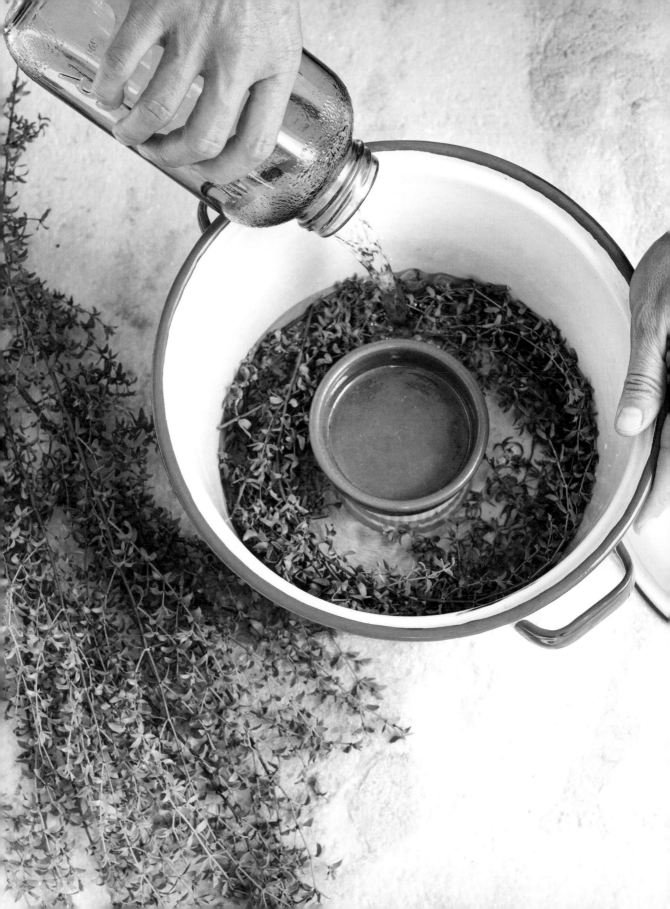

MAKING YOUR OWN HYDROSOLS

Using hydrosols, sometimes referred to as floral waters, is an excellent way to get the aromatic properties of plants into a water-based solution. The aromatic byproduct after the steam-distillation process occurs, hydrosols can be made using simple kitchen equipment. (Note that hydrosols cannot be made by simply adding essential oils to water.) They have been used for centuries in skin tonics, for cooking, or to flavor medicinal cordials. The best-known examples are lavender, orange blossom, and rose waters.

I started making hydrosols when I was living in Seattle and had such homesickness for the desert. It rained all the time in Seattle, but the rain didn't smell like anything to me. I realized it was the scent of Grandmother Creosote, the signature scent of the Sonoran Desert, that I was longing for. The creosote bush releases aromatics during the monsoon rains, emitting a scent that awakens your senses. Whenever I felt homesick, I would spritz my creosote hydrosol around my apartment and instantly feel a little closer to home. By following this method, you will be able to create your own personal hydrosols to use as a cooling body spray, facial mist, or even your own rose water for desserts! When creating your hydrosol, use fresh, organic plant material, not dried, and always use sterile supplies.

Makes about 3½ cups

Fresh herbs or flowers, about 5 cups (see page 40)

4 cups of water, preferably distilled

8-ounce (or larger) dark glass bottle with mister

(continued)

Gather

About 3 or 4 handfuls of one or a mix of the following:

Calendula *is an antibacterial*

Citrus blossoms *uplift the spirits*

Creosote *is an antibacterial*

Lavender *is calming and good for sunburn*

Mint *is good for hot flashes*

Rose petals *are good for hormonal balance*

Rosemary *is uplifting*

The night before starting your hydrosol, fill a large glass mixing bowl with tap water and place it in the freezer. You will have a bowl of solid ice to use the next day to make your hydrosol.

In a large pot, place a heat-resistant ramekin or similar object upside down on the bottom of the pot. Arrange the fresh herbs on the bottom of the pot around the ramekin. Add 4 cups of filtered water to the pot, then place the glass measuring cup on top of the ramekin. This will catch the hydrosol water. Turn the heat on and bring the water to a boil. Once the water reaches a boil, turn the heat down to gently simmer the herbs. Place the entire glass bowl of ice on top of the pot as a lid. This will cool the steam and allow the water droplets to fall into the glass measuring cup. Continue simmering until most of the water from the pot has been turned into a hydrosol and is collected into the glass measuring cup. When finished, allow the hydrosol to cool before pouring it into your glass bottle. Pour the remainder in a glass jar with a tight lid to refill your mister as needed. Label the bottle and jar and store them in the refrigerator.

MINERAL-RICH HAIR MOISTURIZER

I was taught that our hair carries our life force energy as well as our thoughts and memories, so caring for your hair is very important. If you are looking to keep the energy in your hair strong and receptive, it is important that you do not coat your hair with toxic chemicals such as sulfates that can also dry it out. Many years ago, while preparing Irish sea moss (red algae that grows all over the Atlantic coast of Europe and North America) to thicken a dish, I learned I could also apply the gel to my skin as an emollient. It worked wonderfully.

So I decided to experiment with it on my hair and came up with this recipe, which I most often use to braid my hair. I first make the Sea Moss Gel, and then use that as the base for the Life Force Hair Gel. I simply apply the final gel to damp hair, combing it through with good thoughts and prayers, and then braid my hair tightly to keep those thoughts in place. When I unbraid my hair, I have super-soft moisturized waves.

Since it's rich in minerals, you can also play with the Sea Moss Gel recipe first by trying it on your face! It works wonders on helping my skin retain moisture. Just wash your face and apply a little gel to your skin, allow it to dry, then rinse with warm water.

(continued)

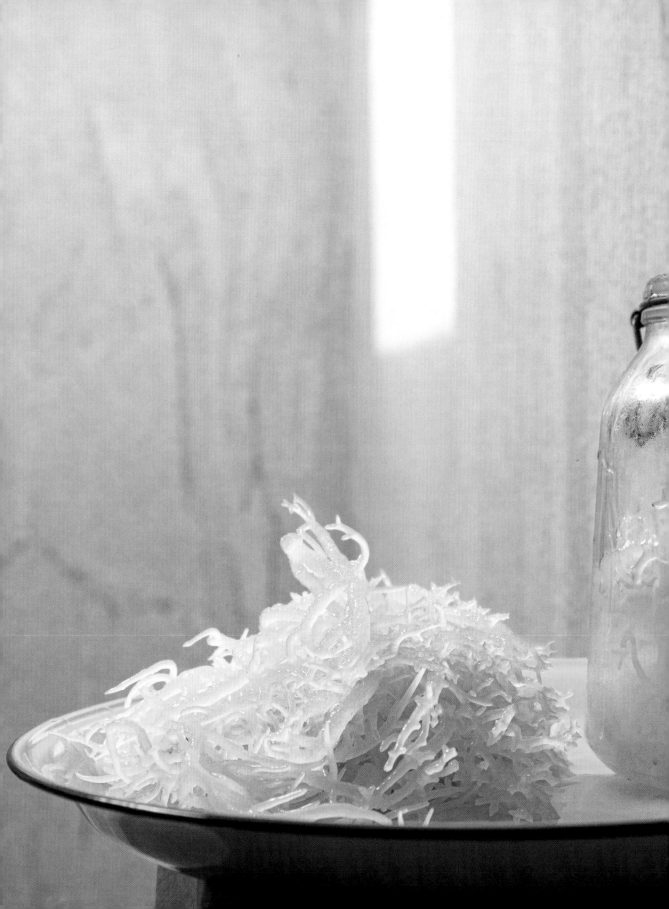

LA SIRENA SEA MOSS GEL

Makes about 1 cup

2 ounces dried organic whole sea moss (see note)
1 cup purified water
8-ounce glass jar

Dried whole sea moss also goes by Irish sea moss and can be found at many Caribbean stores, health food stores, and online.

Rinse the dried sea moss well to remove any debris. After rinsing, place the sea moss in a large bowl and cover it with cool water. Leave the bowl on the counter to soak overnight. The next day, drain the water, place the hydrated sea moss in a blender with the purified water, and puree. The sea moss should be gelatinous in texture. Pour the mixture into a glass jar and store it in the refrigerator.

LIFE FORCE HAIR GEL

Makes about ½ cup

½ cup La Sirena Sea Moss Gel (see above)
¼ cup aloe vera gel (see page 27)
2 tablespoons avocado oil
3 drops neroli essential oil
2 drops geranium essential oil
4-ounce glass jar or squeeze bottle

Add the La Sirena Sea Moss Gel and aloe vera gel to a blender. Blend on low speed, scraping down the sides of the blender with a rubber spatula. Slowly add the avocado oil and blend on low speed until the mixture is well-incorporated. It will be pale white when it's ready. Add the essential oils and pulse a few more times. Pour into a small jar or squeeze bottle. Label and date. I use my gel within a week because I braid my hair often. If you will not be using it that soon, store in the refrigerator and it will keep for up to three weeks.

SIMPLE SEAWEED DETOX MASK

For centuries, people have turned to the sea to harvest seaweed during the low tides of the early mornings. Almost all the minerals found in the Ocean are found in seaweed—such as iodine and magnesium, which can be lacking in most of our diets—making this Ocean plant excellent for your internal and external health. The skin is exposed to a plethora of toxins on a daily basis, and over time, these toxins can take a toll on its health. The rejuvenating effects of seaweed face masks help improve your skin tone and appearance by bringing Ocean nutrients and oxygen to your face while removing impurities from deep inside your pores. This simple, no-mix method results in healthier cells, which in turn helps your skin look more radiant and luminous. When purchasing your dried seaweed, look for a product line that is sourced from clean waters, as seaweed absorbs the seawater in which it lives. In my own home, I only purchase seaweed that is certified organic.

Makes 1 mask

Water
Dried nori seaweed (untoasted, unflavored), torn into enough strips to cover your face

Fill a medium-size bowl with water and place the nori pieces into the bowl, a few strips at a time. The nori will rehydrate almost immediately.

To use the mask, place the strips on your face, avoiding your eyes, nose, and mouth. Keep the mask on your skin for 15 to 20 minutes. Remove the mask and rinse your face. When you're done, compost your seaweed mask, if that is a possibility.

HYDRATING FACE OILS

Natural oils absorb easily into the skin, protecting its lipid barrier and preventing moisture from evaporating out of the skin. The top layer of your skin, called the stratum corneum, is composed of dead skin cells held together by lipids. Keeping this layer constantly supplied with healthy oils will protect your skin and help it have a beautiful, healthy, moisturized glow.

NIGHTTIME HYDRATING FACE OIL

I have been creating this face oil recipe since my early twenties, and I am convinced it has played a key role in how my skin looks today. It is light, perfect for all skin types, and uses jojoba oil as the base, which is an ancestral oil for me. To this base, I add avocado and rose hip seed oils, both wonderful for their nourishing and regenerating properties, and then finish it with frankincense and rose essential oils for their beautiful scents and to support new skin cell growth.

Makes about ¼ cup

3 tablespoons jojoba oil

1 tablespoon avocado oil

2 teaspoons rose hip seed oil

¼ teaspoon vitamin E oil (optional)

4 drops frankincense essential oil

4 drops rose essential oil

2-ounce dark glass bottle with dropper

Using a small funnel, pour the jojoba oil into the dropper bottle. Add the avocado oil, rose hip seed oil, essential oils, and vitamin E oil, if using. Cap the bottle and roll it between your hands to gently blend. Label the bottle and use it within 3 months. To use the face oil, apply ½ to 1 dropperful to clean skin, gently massaging it into your face and neck each evening.

(continued)

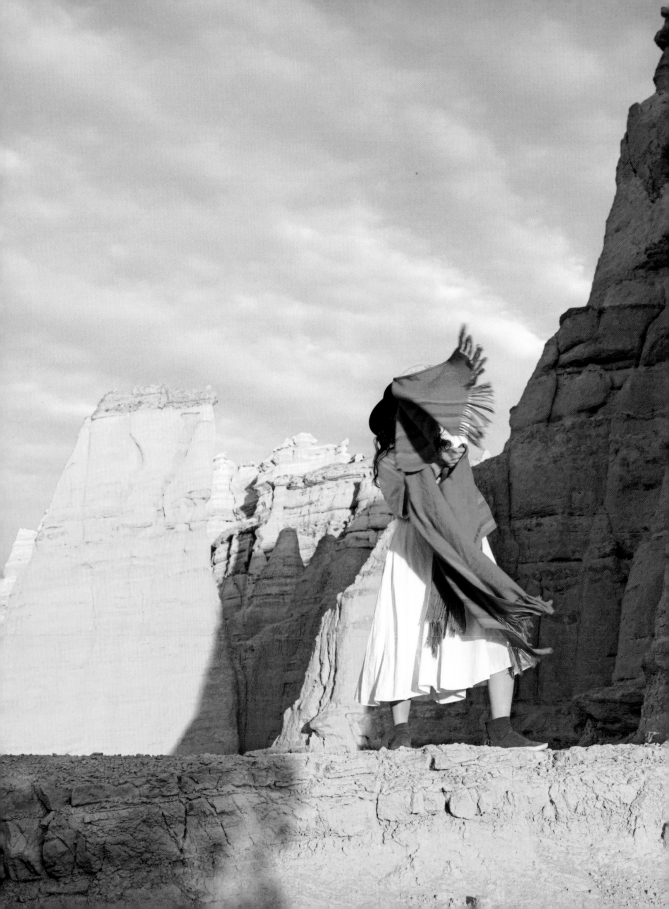

DAYTIME SACRED BEE BALM

For ancient Egyptians, moisturizing emollients were used to protect the skin from the very dry desert climate. For the elite, their oils and unguents would be perfumed with aromatic plants such as cinnamon, pine, and rose. Being a lover of Egyptology and a desert dweller myself, I turned to their creations for inspiration, using ingredients found in their beauty rituals to retain moisture and protect my skin during the day.

Ancient Egyptians loved pleasant-smelling botanicals, and they would use them extensively for perfumes, incense, and medicine along with several oils and fats that are known for their skin-rejuvenating properties. They were also incredible beekeepers, using honey and other bee products in their formulas. I've included frankincense, a known skin restorative, along with beeswax, honey, and royal jelly to create a hydrating face balm for dry environments, including air travel.

Makes about ½ cup

1 teaspoon beeswax pellets

7 teaspoons almond oil

1 teaspoon rose water

¼ teaspoon fine royal jelly powder (1 capsule)

½ teaspoon honey

6 drops frankincense oil

4-ounce glass jar

Add the beeswax, almond oil, and rose water to a double boiler (see page 12) placed on medium-high heat and stir occasionally until the beeswax is melted. Remove the mixture from the heat and immediately add the royal jelly powder, mixing with a whisk. Add the honey and frankincense essential oil, and mix well. Pour the mixture into a glass jar and label. Test the cream on a small area before using. Use a tiny amount whenever you need to hydrate your skin. A little goes a long way.

ORAL HEALTH WITH WATER

Many years ago, while visiting the open-air markets of Aix-en-Provence, France, I fell in love with the abundance of herbs and spices used in everything, from tea blends to shortbread cookies. One tea I truly enjoyed was simply a few dried leaves of common sage infused in water and served with lavender honey. I learned that many of the grandmothers throughout Aix grow and use common sage not only for culinary uses but also for its healing qualities, including its ability to soothe sensitive gums and sore throats.

Here are two alcohol-free mouth rinses created with sage and other herbs and spices that will help keep harmful bacteria in check while soothing gums and protecting tooth enamel.

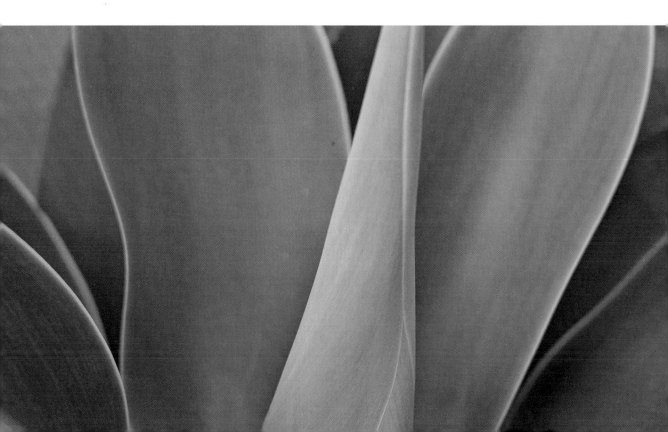

SALTWATER HERBAL MOUTH RINSE

Makes about 1½ cups

1½ cups water

3 teaspoons dried culinary sage

1 teaspoon dried lavender

1 teaspoon fennel seeds

¼ teaspoon anise seeds

½ teaspoon fine sea salt

12-ounce glass jar

Bring water to boil into the small saucepan. Add dried herbs, seeds, and sea salt. Turn off the heat and allow the herbs to infuse for 30 minutes. Strain the cooled mixture into a jar using a funnel lined with the cheesecloth or fine-mesh strainer, label, store in the refrigerator. To use the mouth rinse, swish 1 tablespoon in your mouth for 30 seconds, then spit it out.

SWEETWATER HERBAL MOUTH RINSE

Makes about 1½ cups

1½ cups water

1 handful fresh culinary sage

1 handful fresh mint

1 tablespoon vegetable glycerin

5 drops spearmint or peppermint essential oil

12-ounce glass jar

Bring the water to boil in a small saucepan. Add herbs. Turn the heat off and allow the herbs to infuse for 30 minutes. Once cool, strain the herbal water into a glass measuring cup and stir in the glycerin and essential oil. Using a funnel, pour your mixture into a glass jar, label it, and store it in the refrigerator. To use the mouth rinse, swish 1 tablespoon in your mouth for 30 seconds, then spit it out.

SPIRITUAL WORK WITH WATER

FELICIA'S AGUA DE FLORIDA

Agua de Florida is a fragrant water used for spiritual cleansing, blessing, and protection. It began as a cologne called Florida Water in the early 1800s, and versions were soon adopted by Caribbean, Central American, and South American spiritual workers of all traditions for religious practices. There are countless recipes for Florida Water, which at its core is a combination of alcohol and aromatics. As many store-bought Florida Waters include synthetic fragrances and are sold in plastic bottles, I started making my own, which takes one full lunation to infuse.

I created this recipe using essential oils for times when I needed Florida Water in a pinch. Use it as a base recipe, as it is very flexible as long as you limit your essential oils to 25 drops per every 4-ounce bottle. Feel free to substitute your favorite essential oils or floral waters commonly found in botanicas and herbal shops (see below for some ideas). Don't forget to keep notes on your creation.

Personalize Your Agua de Florida

Chamomile water	Geranium essential oil
Bay laurel water	Grapefruit essential oil
Lavender water	Lime essential oil
Rose water	Jasmine essential oil
Allspice essential oil	Neroli essential oil
Cinnamon essential oil	Ylang-ylang essential oil

(continued)

Makes about ½ cup

Distilled water

2 tablespoons witch hazel extract

5 tablespoons orange blossom water

6 drops orange essential oil

5 drops bergamot essential oil

4 drops lavender essential oil

4 drops rose essential oil

2 drops cinnamon essential oil

2 drops clove essential oil

4-ounce dark glass bottle with mister

Using a funnel, pour distilled water into the glass bottle, filling it halfway. Add the witch hazel extract, orange blossom water, and essential oils. Top off the bottle with distilled water, being careful not to overflow your mixture and to save room for your mister.

Place your mister on the bottle. While holding your bottle in your hands, close your eyes and set an intention for your Florida Water to infuse it with good energy. I like to say something such as: *May this water bring more sweetness into my life and to the others who smell it.* Shake gently and label.

How to Use

Anoint your entryways to bless and protect your home.

Lightly mist your pillow to ensure good dreams.

Wipe down your altar or sacred space.

Add a splash to your bathwater to spiritually cleanse yourself.

Have it on hand when you need a quick spiritual uplifting.

Add a splash to your mop water to energetically cleanse your home.

ALKALINE SPIRITUAL BATH

Ritual bathing using flowers, herbs, minerals, and oils has been passed down through the generations in many traditions to spiritually purify, attract blessings, or give protection. There are as many botanical blends as there are ideas on how to take a spiritual bath, but my suggestions are to simply be in good spirits when creating your blend and to set a clear intention before stepping into your bathwater.

This recipe includes ingredients to nourish your spiritual and physical well-being by including baking soda, which when added to your ritual bath creates alkaline water and leaves your skin feeling silky soft.

Makes enough for 5 baths

1 cup dried rosebuds or rose petals

1 cup dried calendula flowers

1 cup coarse sea salt

1 cup Epsom salt

½ cup baking soda

½ cup carrier oil such as almond, olive, or sesame

5 drops lavender essential oil

5 sticks of cinnamon

5 star anises

Five 5-by-7-inch muslin bags

In a medium bowl, gently mix together the rose, calendula, sea salt, Epsom salt, baking soda and then slowly mix in the oils. Fill each muslin bag with a cinnamon stick, a star anise, and 1 cup of the blend. Close the bags and store them in a large glass jar. To use your bath blend, add one bag to warm bathwater, squeezing the bag to release the aromatics and energy. If you do not have a bathtub, you can steep the bag in a large pot of hot water, allow it to cool, then pour it over your body while standing in your shower.

OCEAN DEVOTION

Many years ago, I started playing and learning about the Afro-Brazilian martial art called Capoeira Angola. Born from the oppression of slavery, Capoeira Angola is a fluid form of movement often seen as one-part martial art and one-part dance. Knowing I had West African ancestors in my bloodline, this practice allowed me to connect to those ancestors.

Through its songs, Capoeira Angola carries an oral tradition of ancestral wisdom, freedom, and spirituality. In learning the songs (which are sung in Portuguese), I learned about Yemaya. She is the Goddess of the Ocean and is known by different name variations among Afro-Caribbean spiritual traditions. She is one of my favorite deities. Ruler of the sea, the moon, and dreams, many devotees present her with offerings for blessings and gratitude. She is very powerful and is concerned with every aspect of womanhood, reminding women to nurture their own needs and to respect their deserved position in life.

This ritual was designed to honor Yemaya, which in turn, honors and teaches you to listen to yourself. If you do not live near or cannot visit the Ocean, you can prepare a bowl of water sprinkled with sea salt and make adjustments.

Prepare for the Water ritual by first collecting an offering of small shells or white flowers. You want to offer the Ocean some materials that will not harm or pollute her in any way. Next, find a jar or bottle to collect seawater and then head to the Ocean.

When you get to the beach, center yourself in the sand by creating an intention for being there. Think about what you wish to release to the Ocean and what wisdom you wish to receive.

(continued)

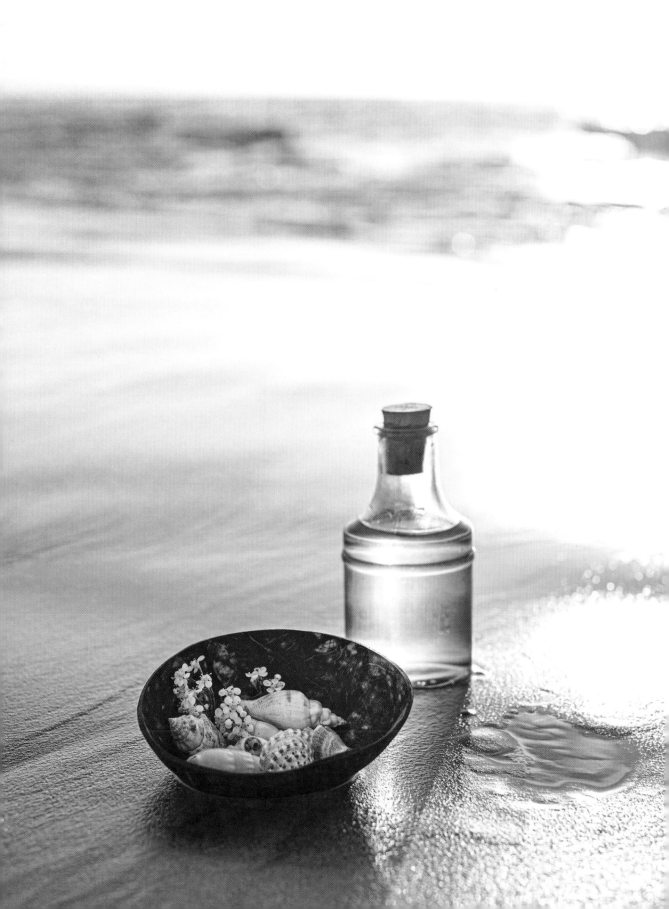

Walk down to the water with your offering and tell Yemaya your intention for being there. Offer her gratitude for listening and then release your offering to her waters. Take a moment to simply listen to the sound of the water and what it has to say. This can be an emotional experience for some, so take your time and allow your own saltwater to flow from your eyes if necessary. They too are making an offering. When you're ready, collect some seawater in your jar or bottle to take home to use later for the Ocean Bath Blessing.

I recommend having a journal with you so that you can write down any feelings, guidance, or pings you felt during your ritual.

OCEAN BATH BLESSING RITUAL

Seawater collected from the previous ritual
Several 2-ounce glass bottles
Bottom-shelf vodka

Fill your jars or bottles about ¾ full with seawater. Top them off with vodka as a preservative. Label your creation. When you feel the call or need to connect with the waters of the Ocean, draw yourself a relaxing bath and empty one bottle of your blessing water into the bathwater, adding a few seashells if you have them for good measure.

MAYAN BAJO STEAMING RITUAL

A Mayan Bajo is a respected treatment using plants and steam, practiced by Mayan women. It can be used to support one's reproductive system and also as a symbolic cleansing ritual after trauma. Herbs and flowers are first simmered in a pot of water, where the essence of their healing properties release into the steam. The woman receiving the treatment then squats over the pot of simmered herbs so the steam can penetrate into her cervix and uterus, where the warmth of the steam is not only relaxing but also increases blood and lymph flow to the area. This ancient practice of using healing steam has been used in many Indigenous cultures across the world to treat numerous conditions including cysts, fibroids, or to support postpartum healing. It's a beautiful ritual that can be done in the privacy of your own home and can also be practiced as preventative care even if you have no chronic issues or trauma.

There are endless herbal combinations to create bajo blends using dried and fresh herbs. I do not suggest or recommend using essential oils in their place, as I believe they are too concentrated for this purpose. Never do vaginal steams when you are pregnant unless you are full-term and under the guidance of your midwife. It is also recommended to avoid steaming while experiencing an active infection, if you are actively bleeding, or use an intrauterine device (IUD).

As this traditional treatment becomes more widespread, women are investing in special steam chairs and stools made for this purpose. However, if you are able to get into the yoga posture child's pose or into a squatting position, all you need is you.

(continued)

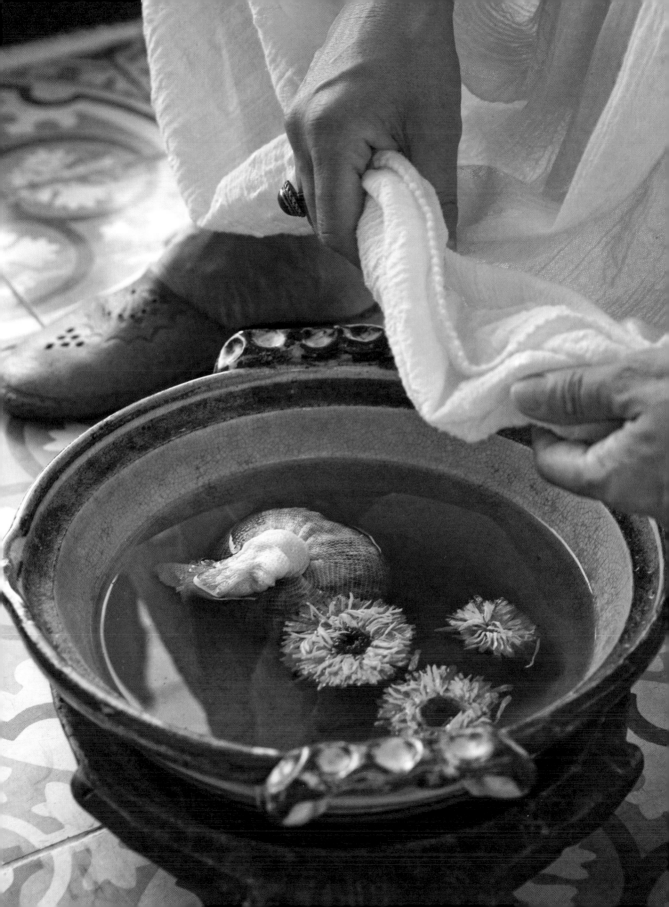

GENTLE HERB BLEND

You will first need to prepare the herbal blend. I have included a recipe of herbs that are nourishing and gentle for women of any age.

Makes enough for 3 steaming rituals

¼ cup dried calendula flowers

¼ cup dried lavender flowers

¼ cup dried lemon balm leaves

½ cup dried red raspberry leaf

¼ cup dried rose petals

12-ounce glass jar

In a large bowl, mix the herbs with your hands, infusing the blend with your good energy. Place your herb blend in the glass jar, seal tightly, and label.

Large handful Gentle Herb Blend (see above)

8 cups water

Beach towel or blanket

Warm socks

Steaming chair or stool (optional)

In a large pot on the stovetop, bring the herbs and water to a boil. Once boiling, cover the pot with the lid and turn the heat down to gently simmer the herbs for 10 minutes, then turn off the heat and infuse the herbs for another 5 minutes. Next, carefully remove the pot from the stove and place it on the floor (protecting the floor with the towel, if needed) to a quiet space.

Remove your clothes from the waist down, or wear a long skirt and no underwear, whichever is most comfortable. Be sure to wear socks to keep your body warm. Slowly release the steam from the pot by removing the lid about one inch. Wrap your blanket or beach towel over your lower body and then check the temperature of the steam on your wrist before carefully positioning yourself over the pot by sitting in child's pose, squatting, or using a steam chair. If the steam is too hot, allow the mixture to cool down slightly. Keep under the blanket with the steam for no more than 20 minutes, releasing more steam midway by moving the lid another inch. Afterward, try to stay warm by resting inside and keeping away from cold drafts.

HONORING YOUR MONTHLY MOON: CASTOR OIL RITUAL

By nature, women's menstrual cycles have long been associated with the moon. A woman's cycle is commonly the same as a lunar month, whose own energy is tied to the energy of Water through the low and high tides of the Ocean. Our moontime is considered sacred and powerful for women, as we are able to purify our bodies each cycle by releasing any negative energies we may be carrying. Supporting this process with castor oil not only helps us detox but also reminds us to slow down and honor our wombs and its energy.

Castor oil packs have been used in many cultures around the world for the many benefits they provide, including moontime support. Made from the castor bean, castor oil helps release toxins from the pelvic area while stimulating the natural cleansing process of the tissues. For general womb health, you can use castor oil packs every day, pausing while you are actively bleeding. Castor oil packs are considered very safe but are contraindicated during pregnancy or if you use an intrauterine device (IUD). Please talk to your health care provider before using if you have cancerous fibroids or ovarian tumors.

Cotton flannel, 3 layers thick, about 1 square foot in size
Castor oil
Old towel
Plastic wrap or plastic bag
Hot water bottle or electric heating pad

Put your cotton flannel in a mixing bowl and then pour castor oil onto the fabric until it is saturated. You now have a castor oil pack. Place the old towel on the floor or bed and lay down on it. Place the castor oil pack on your abdominal area. Cover the pack with the plastic wrap or bag. Place the hot water bottle or electric heating pad (set on low–medium) on top of the plastic layer. Rest in place for up to one hour, then remove the castor oil pack and gently massage any remaining oil in a clockwise motion.

You can store the castor oil pack in a glass container to be used again. The same pack can be used 2 to 3 times. Castor oil packs can be used as a weekly ritual or as needed to help relieve stagnation in the pelvic region.

HEALING SPRING WATER

There are many hot springs scattered throughout Northern New Mexico that are believed by my Tewa ancestors to be special gifts from Creator. The springs are thought to be a portal between this world and the world below. Hot springs are found where volcanic activity is present or where there are fault lines in the Earth. Their high mineral content and geothermal water are believed to soothe aching muscles, aid arthritis, help circulation, and more. But it's the spiritual aspect I love most. Relaxing in a hot spring fosters a sense of overall centeredness because while soaking, we are virtually holding space where the two worlds meet.

Drinking water from a natural spring is another experience I partake in, as there is a spring not too far from my home where I can collect water by the gallon. The water has a slight mineral taste that almost feels slippery on my tongue and is far more refreshing than water I can get at the water mart. All spring water contains trace minerals, so it carries with it the Earth. To consume it as medicine is one of the best ways to spiritually connect with Water.

(continued)

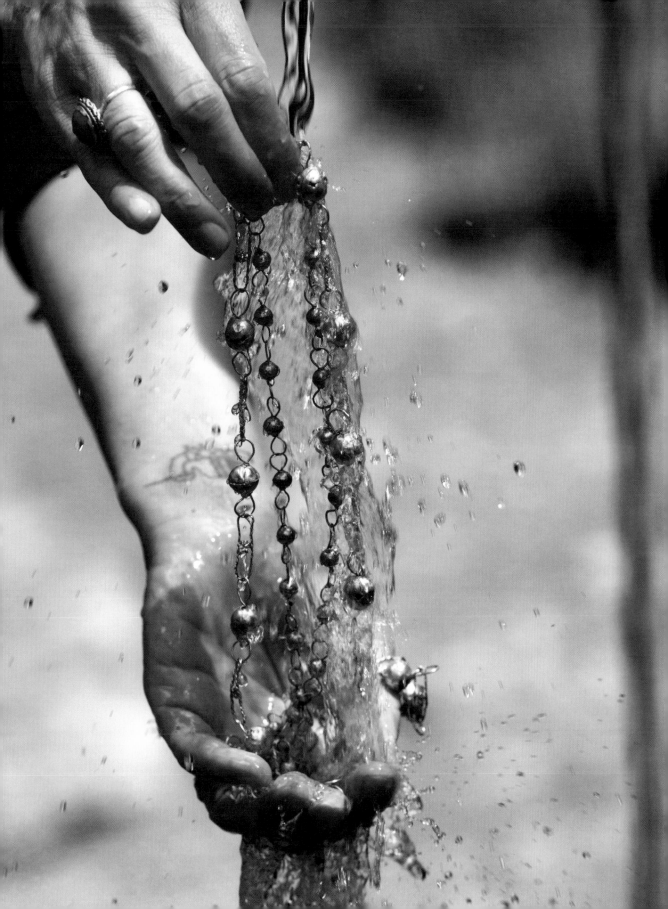

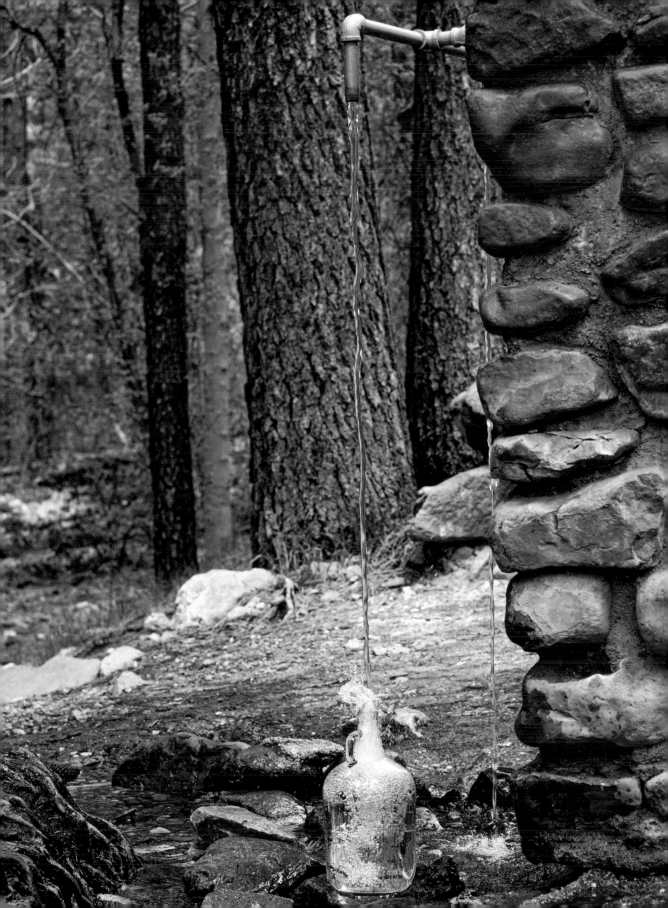

RELAXING IN THE HOT SPRINGS

Wild or resort? Hot springs exist all over the world, many still in their wild state and others now on resort properties. I've been to both, and it just depends on what type of experience you are looking for. The major difference between the two is that resort hot springs must comply with various health standards for water quality, while there is generally no agency that monitors the cleanliness of natural wild springs. Before soaking in a hot spring, here are a few things to take into account:

- Take off your jewelry before entering.
- If you are pregnant, have a heart condition, or have any other health concerns, check with your health care or birth care provider first.
- Never put your head underwater in a wild hot spring.
- Keep hydrated and avoid alcohol prior to soaking.

DRINKING SPRING WATER

Natural springs, which generally form alongside hills and mountain valleys, come from an underground source where water rises naturally to the surface. Flowing through the ground, the water picks up trace minerals like calcium, magnesium, and potassium along the way, which I believe is what makes it taste so good. I often hear from people who are nervous to drink water from a roadside source, so I wanted to share what I do, so you can make your own decision. Here are a few tips for collecting spring water to drink:

- Look around to be certain that groundwater is coming out of a spigot versus being piped in from a stream or river.
- Check around the spring to see if there is any debris or waste that could affect the water.
- Look for signage that says the spring gets regularly tested. If it is, test results will be on file.
- Have the water tested yourself.
- Many people stopping to collect water at a spring is a *good* indication that it is safe to drink!

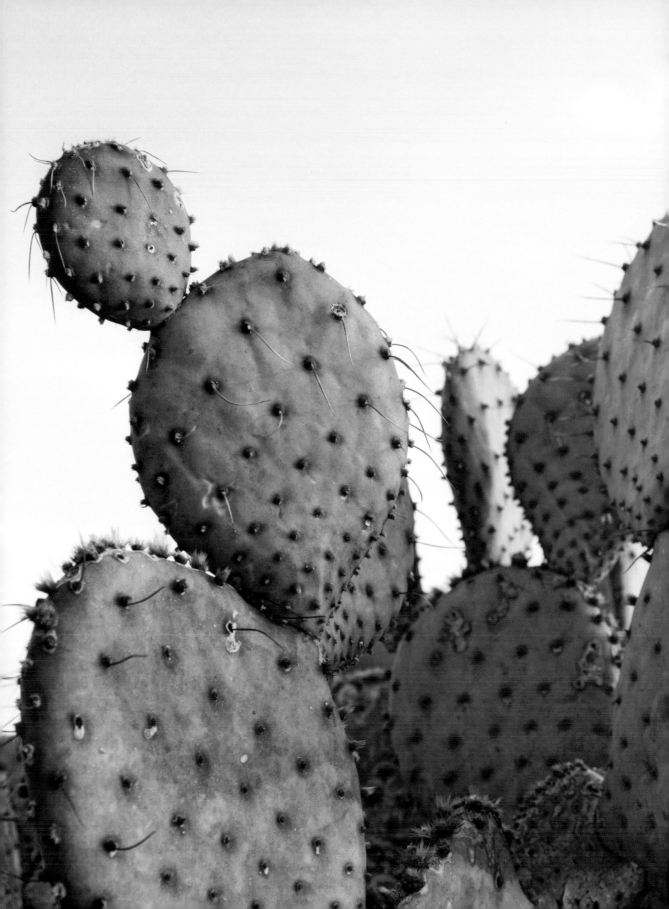

67 ◇ AIR

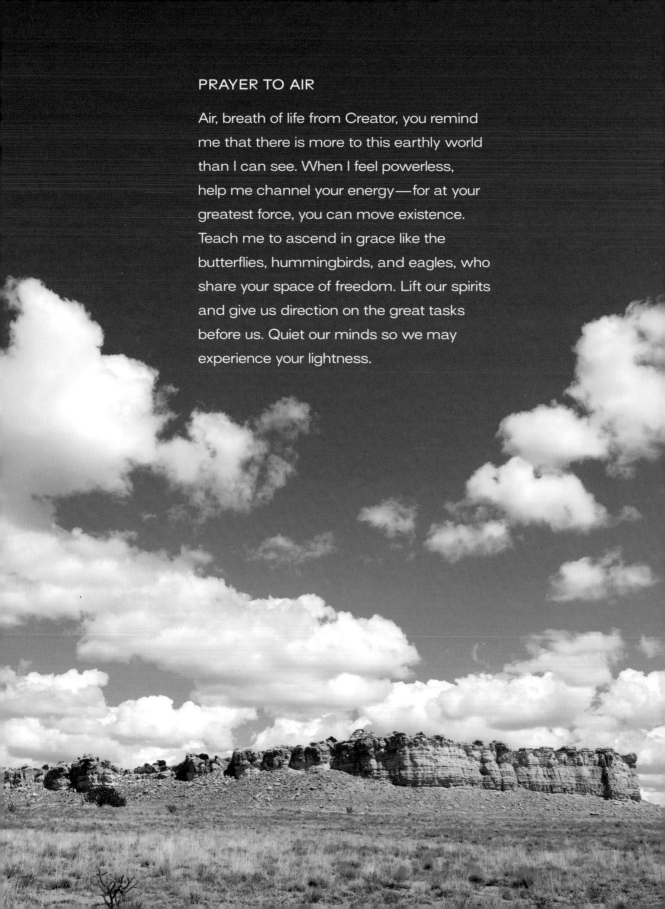

PRAYER TO AIR

Air, breath of life from Creator, you remind
me that there is more to this earthly world
than I can see. When I feel powerless,
help me channel your energy—for at your
greatest force, you can move existence.
Teach me to ascend in grace like the
butterflies, hummingbirds, and eagles, who
share your space of freedom. Lift our spirits
and give us direction on the great tasks
before us. Quiet our minds so we may
experience your lightness.

AIR FOR INNER HARMONY

THE BEAUTY OF AIR

SPIRITUAL WORK WITH AIR

AIR REPRESENTS FREEDOM, MOVEMENT, AND DIRECTION

When its energy is subtle, I like the way it moves my hair and makes my whole essence feel carefree. Its personality at this intensity reminds me of my childhood, playing outside moments before the desert rains began. The scented wind would lure us outside, telling us that rain was on its way. We would feel it and breathe it in. However, when its personality turns forceful, different feelings trigger, urging us to go inside and take shelter. The wind tells us that change is coming. Air has a superpower that the other elements do not possess: it can carry the other elements, working as a messenger. Our bodies are in constant contact with Air, absorbing all its strengths and particles throughout the day. Immersed in its invisible magic, our skin reminds us of the cycle of life with the growth and death of its cells.

Ehécatl is the Aztec/Mexica metaphorical representation of wind. His name means "wind" in Nahuatl, and he is regarded as one of the many faces of the beautiful serpent Quetzalcoatl in our Creation stories. Ehécatl is depicted in many ancient art pieces wearing a conch shell (*ehecailacocozcatl* or "wind jewel") on his chest that he uses to blow the world into motion. I believe there is much creative energy behind the motion of the wind and, when we are in the midst of wind's presence, we are sensing intuitive direction or awareness. Our own breath is wind birthing our intentions, affirmations, gratitude, and desires. However, sometimes we need assistance in speaking these truths. Air can be used as a tool to encourage a focused mind and receive mental clarity by awakening vibrations in our bodies that encourage clear communication. Having heightened intuition, using your voice, opening your throat chakra—these are all benefits you can receive from working with the element of Air.

Physically, being outside in fresh Air has been shown to improve blood pressure, strengthen the immune system, and help the airways of the lungs to dilate more fully, improving their cleansing action. Most of the time, we are more aware of the Air in our immediate environment than the Air in our bodies. We may see a haze of pollution in the distance, sense stagnant Air in a closed space, or feel crisp Air during a morning walk. We tend to think of Air as being outside of us. Truth is, there are no defined boundaries with Air. As you read this, Air is entering your body, oxygen is flowing into your bloodstream, and carbon dioxide is being exhaled back into the Air you just took in. Our bodies simply borrow this life-giving element for a brief moment before it returns to its place of abundance. How beautiful it is that we have made this agreement!

Emotionally speaking, simply being outside in fresh Air fosters positive emotions and betters our ability to handle stress. I encourage you to get outside at least once a day or simply open a window if weather permits, and breathe in this element of awareness.

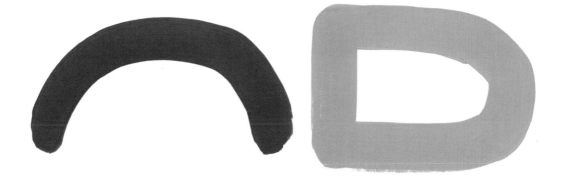

AIR FOR
INNER
HARMONY

LUNG SUPPORT INFUSIONS

The ability to breathe is something we often take for granted. Often, it's not until we are experiencing a cold or are working through an asthma attack that we are reminded how precious it is to take in a long, deep breath. Our lungs' purpose is to filter out contaminants from the air and bring in life-giving oxygen so that we may live. In exchange, we exhale carbon dioxide to be used by our plant relatives, working together symbiotically.

Since our lungs work as filters, they are very susceptible to infections. We can support them during times of respiratory despair with the help of herbal lung-openers. One of my favorite go-to herbs for lung support is the needles from the piñon pine tree, a high-desert evergreen that is native to Arizona and New Mexico. My family has used piñon pine for food, healing, and in spiritual practices as it's known for its vibrational properties.

These aromatic teas are antimicrobial, soothing, and wonderful for chest congestion. When the piñon releases its balsam-like scent, it reminds me of summers when I visit relatives near Taos and Santa Fe, the *tierra adentro*, the far land.

(continued)

PIÑON NEEDLE TEA

Makes about 2 cups

Handful fresh green pine needles, rinsed
2 cups water
Natural sweetener (honey or maple syrup)

Mince the pine needles using a sharp knife or a pair of kitchen scissors. Set aside. Bring the water to boil in a small saucepan or teakettle. Place about 2 tablespoons of the minced needles in a tea infuser, tea bag, or French press. Pour the boiling water over the needles and infuse for 15 minutes. Strain, add your sweetener of choice to taste, and enjoy.

DESERT DEW LUNG SUPPORT TEA

Makes 2 cups of the herbal blend

You can easily adapt the yield of this recipe to suit your needs by measuring equal amounts of each herb.

For the blend:
¼ cup fresh green pine needles, rinsed and minced
¼ cup dried bee balm
¼ cup dried yerba santa
¼ cup dried spearmint
8-ounce glass jar

For the tea:
Natural sweetener (honey or maple syrup)

Mince the needles using a sharp knife or a pair of kitchen scissors. Add all the herbs to a small bowl and mix to combine. Put the blend in the glass jar and label.

To make the tea, use 1 tablespoon of the blend per each cup (about 8 ounces) of water. Bring the water to a boil in a small saucepan or teakettle. Place your desired amount of the herbal mixture in a tea infuser, tea bag, or French press. Pour boiling water over the herbs and infuse for 15 minutes. Strain, add your sweetener of choice to taste, and enjoy.

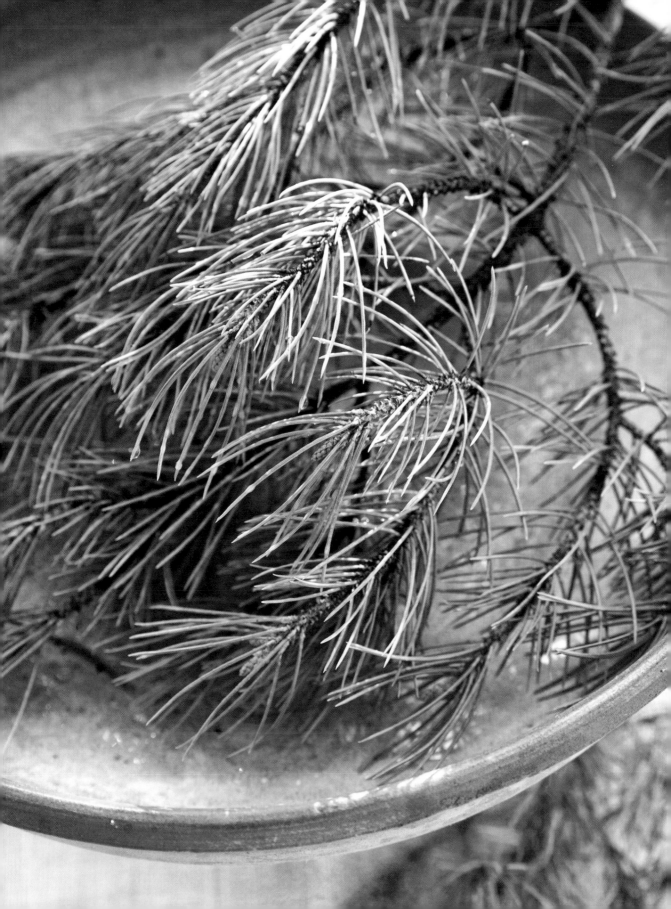

THE FOURTH SISTER: SUNFLOWER MICROGREENS

As an indigenous foods activist, many of my teachings revolve around the Three Sisters: corn, beans, and squash. Corn, beans, and squash are in many of our oral stories and have been cultivated together for generations for their ability to get along so well as plant relatives. The cornstalk acts as a trellis for the beans, which makes nitrogen more available for the soil by cultivating beneficial bacteria. Meanwhile, the squash's wide leaves carpet the earth, preventing weed growth and loss of soil moisture. Not only do these three sisters grow well together, but they are also nutritionally complete, offering a mix of fiber, protein, and natural sugars.

However, there is one *other* sister that is oftentimes left out, and I feel she is just as valuable: the sunflower. All the many varieties of sunflowers are indigenous to North America and have been cultivated for food and medicine in many tribes. Sunflowers are one of my favorite flowers, especially *Helianthus annuus*, the ones with the big, round faces. The seeds are delicious and nutritious when eaten raw or roasted, but it's the microgreens that hold all the chlorophyll, which harnesses the sun's ultraviolet light. It is believed that chlorophyll is the life force of a plant, which may help increase the flow of oxygen throughout your body. Chlorophyll in sunflower microgreens and other greens helps in neutralizing the pollution we breathe in every day.

Growing your own sunflower microgreens in your home is relatively easy as you can purchase sunflower seeds at most grocery stores in the bulk bins. Just be certain they are not roasted so they germinate. There are many methods to grow sunflower microgreens, but this is one of my favorites because it's small enough to have in my tiny kitchen.

Amount varies

1 cup raw sunflower seeds, in the shell
Potting soil
2 pie pans
Spray bottle of water

Soak your sunflower seeds overnight in tap water and drain them the next day. Set aside. Fill one pie pan with about an inch of potting soil. Sow your seeds evenly across the whole tray. You do not need to cover your sunflower seeds with soil. Just be certain they are gently pressed down, so they make contact with the soil. Use the spray bottle to mist the seeds and soil so they are moist. Nest the second pie pan on top of the seed pan so it gently rests on the soil. Place your seeds in a dark space such as a closet or pantry.

Each day, lift your pie pan cover and mist the seeds to keep them moist. You don't want them soaking wet. After 4 or 5 days, take off the top pie pan and allow the seedlings to be exposed to sunlight by placing them near a bright window for 8 or more hours per day. They will quickly turn bright green, and from this point, you can water the soil directly rather than misting. Your sunflower microgreens will be ready to harvest in about 10 days, depending on the conditions. They will be about 4 inches tall.

Harvesting Your Microgreens

The easiest way to harvest your greens is with scissors. Simply trim the most mature greens just above the soil level, leaving the immature ones to grow another day or two. If you see some of the shells still attached to the microgreens, simply remove the shell. And if you're lucky, you may be able to get a second round of microgreens! After you harvest your microgreens, rinse them gently and store them between a moistened towel. Keep them in the refrigerator in a glass container. They will last for up to 5 days stored this way.

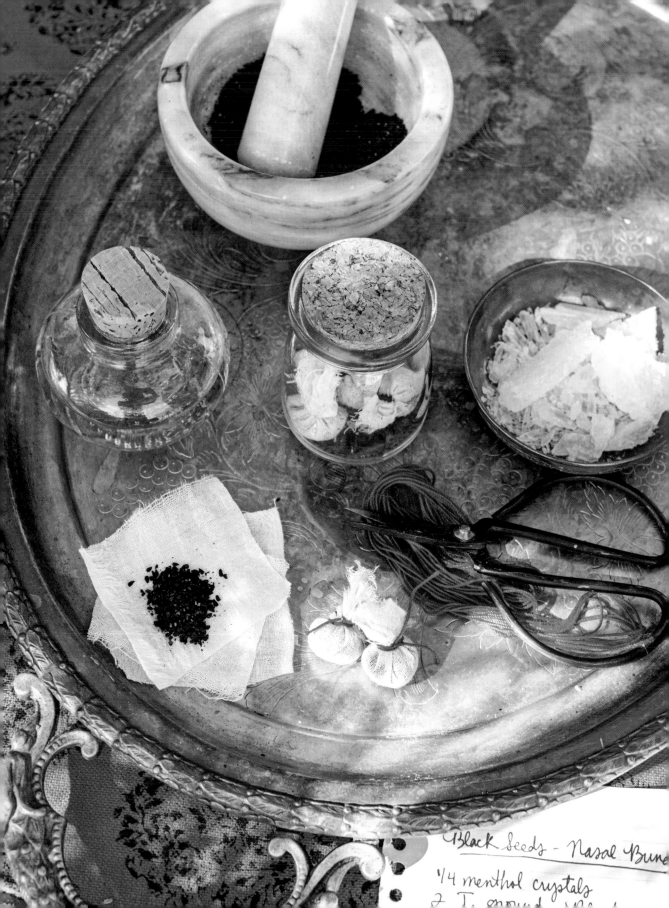

Black Seeds - Nasal Bun

1/4 menthol crystals

BLACK SEED NASAL BUNDLES

The air-filled cavities of your sinuses can become infected, causing pain and inflammation resulting in sinusitis. I myself have suffered from terrible sinusitis during the changing of seasons, creating pressure in my face and pain in my teeth.

As a medicine maker, I love learning other herbalist' traditional healing ways, and this remedy is based on knowledge shared by my friend Lamisa, who is originally from Iraq. She eats black seeds (*Nigella sativa*) with honey as an immune system tonic the moment she begins to feel under the weather or inhales their aromatics when she feels a sinus headache coming. Black seeds work wonderfully to relieve sinus-headache pain due to their natural anti-histaminic effect. This means that they help your ability to breathe by reducing the inflammation of the sinuses and respiratory airways that is triggered by the body's histamine response. Experimenting with their aromatics, I created these potent little bundles to inhale on the go.

Makes about 10 bundles

2 tablespoons ground black seeds

¼ teaspoon organic menthol crystals

5 drops oregano essential oil

Muslin cloth cut into 2-by-2-inch squares

Thread

If your black seeds are not ground, you first need to grind them using a mortar and pestle until you have 2 ground tablespoons. To your ground black seeds, add the menthol crystals and grind again until you have a fine powder. Next, add the oregano essential oil and mix it with a small spoon. Place one square of your muslin

(continued)

cloth on your workstation and add one small spoonful of the black seed mixture to the center of your square. Pinch your square together to create a small bundle, and then tie it closed with a piece of thread. Repeat this procedure until the mixture is used up. Keep the bundles in a glass container labeled with the date.

To use your bundles, take out one bundle and breathe in its aroma when you feel the need to open your airways.

ROSEMARY TONIC FOR COLD AIR

Many of us with Mexican ancestry were told as children to protect our heads from *el Viento*, the wind, especially if it was a cold wind. This belief stems from our traditional folk medicine, which is deeply rooted in humoral concepts of "hot" and "cold." Cold air is believed to have the ability to penetrate our bodies, affecting our joints and causing arthritis, rheumatism, or even headaches. This was reinforced in one of my plant outings when I was collecting plants with a Yaqui elder in the dry desert of February. While collecting plants, a cold blast of wind swept through our area, tangling up our skirts and throwing sand into our faces. The first thing she did was place her scarf over her head, and then she signaled me to do the same. Although I should have known better, I wasn't wearing one, nor did I have one in my bag. I was, however, wearing an apron, so she made me take off the apron and put it over my head before we headed back inside.

Personally, when I feel cold wind in my ears, I experience pain that lasts a few hours. And as I creep into my elder years, cold environments also make my body feel a little achy until it warms up. To help with cold joints, I learned a simple traditional Mexican remedy that uses rubbing alcohol and rosemary. Many Mexican grandmothers made home remedios using rubbing alcohol combined with different herbs, and because rosemary is considered a warming herb, it is applied to help bring heat to our joints. This rosemary tonic is useful after you have spent time in el Viento. Instead of using rubbing alcohol, I have substituted a bottom-shelf vodka.

Makes about 4 cups

1–1½ cups fresh rosemary, chopped (leaves and stems)
4 cups bottom-shelf vodka
1-quart glass jar

Put the chopped rosemary in the jar and cover it with vodka. Place the lid on the jar and label it. Put your jar in a cool, dark cupboard for at least 1 month. After 1 month, you can strain the mixture or use it straight from the jar.

To use, pour a spoonful into your hands and massage it into your muscles and joints to stimulate circulation.

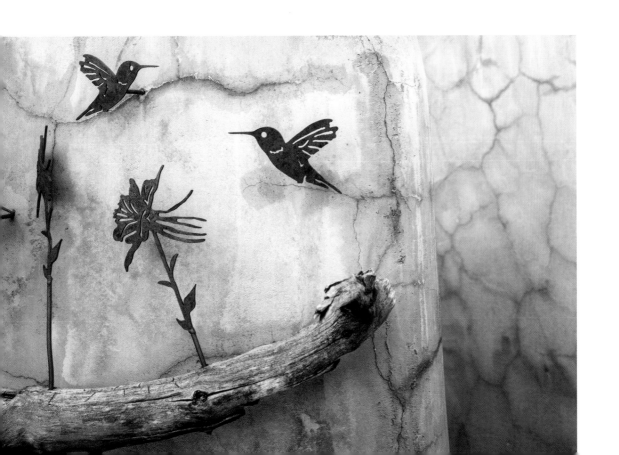

TWENTY FLOWER OIL

Cempaxochitl (*Tagetes erecta*), also known as Mexican marigold, is a sacred flower probably known to most for its use during Day of the Dead celebrations. Its apple-like scent is used to call the ancestors back to Earthside during our Día de los Muertos celebrations, where they are displayed on our altars on this special night. Meaning "twenty flower" in Nahuatl, cempaxochitl has brightly colored, starlike petals that have long been used in ceremony and medicine in Mexico, where they grow wild. As a medicine, cempaxochitl is used for digestive ailments and wounds as well as respiratory complaints such as sinus congestion.

I was originally working on an anointing blend to be used as a tool to connect with ancestors during Día de los Muertos. But when working with the flower and bottling up the blend, I found the stuffy nose I had was gone, which made sense because cempaxochitl is a decongestant. This simple recipe uses *Tagetes erecta* essential oil and Indian sesame oil, which is found in many Ayurvedic nasal treatments. The oil will lubricate your mucous membranes, helping to decongest your nose so you can breathe more freely. The blend is highly diluted from the original anointing blend as its intention is to be used in your sinus passages; however, you can still dab it on your wrists and temples when calling on your ancestors. This truly is plantcestor medicine!

Makes about 5 milliliters

Untoasted sesame oil
1 drop cempaxochitl essential oil (*Tagetes erecta*)
5 milliliter dark glass bottle with dropper

Fill the bottle about ⅔ full of sesame oil. Add the cempaxochitl essential oil. Top off the bottle with more sesame oil, saving a little space for your dropper. Shake gently.

To use your flower oil, instill 1 or 2 drops of oil in your nose and wait at least an hour to see how you feel. The mucous membranes are very delicate, hence the very low dilution. If this strength suits you, label your creation and use it when needed. If you are not having any sensitivity to the blend and would like it slightly stronger, simply add one more drop of the essential oil.

TREE MEDICINE BREATHING BARS

Trees' needles, leaves, and resins has long been used in traditional healing for several ailments, both physical and spiritual. Much tree medicine is specifically for respiratory complaints and help with opening up breathing passageways. Copaiba resin (*Copaifera officinalis*), which is harvested from the trunk of trees that are indigenous to Central and South America, has been found effective in enhancing respiratory capacity, allowing one to breathe in air more freely. In my own family, we work with *Pinus edulis*, which goes by many names such as Colorado piñon pine. Virtually every part of this tree is medicine to us. If you cannot source Colorado piñon pine, you can substitute the more common pine essential oil, Scots pine (*Pinus sylvestris*), which shares the same qualities.

This therapeutic breathing bar incorporates a high dilution of essential oils, meaning it is not to be used continuously,

(continued)

but only during times of respiratory distress. I created this combination years ago when I felt compelled to help friends who were complaining of breathing issues during one of the many California wildfires. As their forests were burning and their lungs were compromised, it was still the trees that were providing medicine. Breathe in the tree medicine deeply as needed and know you are also anointing your body with a scent of protection.

Makes about 3 small lotion bars (about 6 ounces)

2 ounces beeswax pellets

2 ounces raw shea butter

2 ounces avocado oil

30 drops copaiba essential oil

25 drops frankincense essential oil

20 drops green myrtle essential oil

20 drops pine essential oil

Silicone molds totaling 6 ounces

Place the beeswax, shea butter, and avocado oil in the top half of a double boiler (see page 12). Add water to the bottom half and place the whole boiler on the stove. Turn heat to medium. Once the water is simmering and the mixture has melted, remove from heat. Cool slightly, then add the essential oils to the melted mixture and stir. Pour your mixture into the silicone molds. Allow the bars to set and then transfer to the refrigerator or freezer until you're ready to use them. To use, hold the lotion bar in your hands and warm it with your body heat. This will melt a small portion of the bar, allowing you to smooth it over your chest area.

Other Tree Oils Beneficial for Respiratory Issues

Cajeput

Atlas Cedarwood

Balsam Fir

Blue Spruce

Eucalyptus

Hong Kuai

Juniper Berry

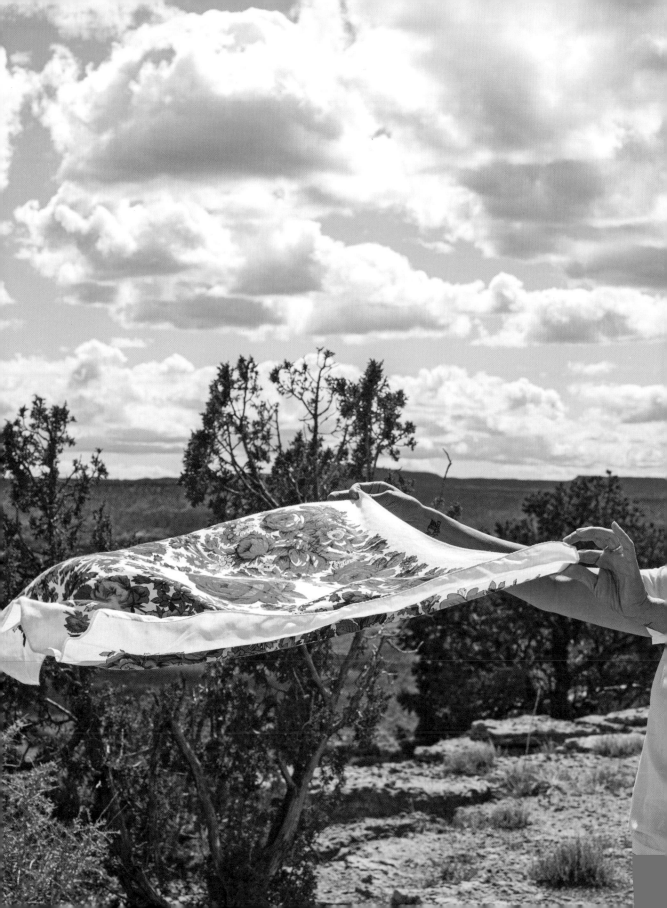

THE BEAUTY OF AIR

CROWN CHAKRA DRY SHAMPOO

Everyone has some degree of intuition, an inner guidance system stemming from the crown chakra, which provides us with a constant flow of information and insight. When your crown chakra is fully open, it enables you to connect with your Higher Self. You may be asking yourself, *What does intuition have to do with dry shampoo?* Well, this is where alchemy really happens in my world, combining the physical with the spiritual.

We have all heard in some context that a woman's crown is her hair. I combined the physical with the spiritual to create a dry shampoo that, when sprinkled on my crown chakra, not only leaves my scalp oil–free and smelling magical but also awakens my intuition.

This recipe uses arrowroot powder, which is great for my silver-colored hair. If you have very dark-colored hair, try substituting a tablespoon or two of cacao powder for arrowroot powder to darken it up a bit.

Makes about ⅓ cup

6 tablespoons arrowroot powder

2 drops rosemary essential oil

2 drops basil essential oil

2 drops Atlas cedarwood oil

2 drops frankincense essential oil

4-ounce glass jar or bottle

Mix all the ingredients in a bowl with a spoon. Store the dry shampoo in the glass jar with a label. To use your powder, dip a makeup brush into the jar and dust a small amount of the powder on the roots of your hair, your crown chakra. Use your fingers, a brush, or a comb to distribute the powder evenly through your hair, embracing your inner knowing.

CORN WOMAN
FACIAL SCRUB

Corn Woman is one of the most important deities in our Pueblo stories. Synonymous with Mother Earth herself, she represents growth, life, and all things feminine. Blue cornmeal mush was one of the first foods I ate as a young child, and it is something I still enjoy when I crave something comforting. I carry blue cornmeal with me for offerings and protection, and its scent alone is one of my absolute favorites.

Living in a large city with air pollutants in the form of dust, carbon monoxide, and soot, can affect the health of your skin, clogging its pores and accumulating on its surface. I like to bring new growth and life to my face by using blue cornmeal as an air pollution remover. Finely ground blue cornmeal gently removes dead skin cells and promotes healthy skin cell growth. I use this scrub in the evening, especially after a long day outside in the city.

Makes 1 facial scrub

¼ cup finely ground blue cornmeal
1 teaspoon aloe vera gel (see page 27)
1 teaspoon runny honey
1 drop lavender essential oil

In a small dish, mix all the ingredients into a paste. To use your scrub, use your fingertips to apply to damp skin. Rub it into your skin, gently exfoliating in circular motions. Rinse with warm water and pat dry. If you have any remaining scrub, store it in a small jar in the refrigerator.

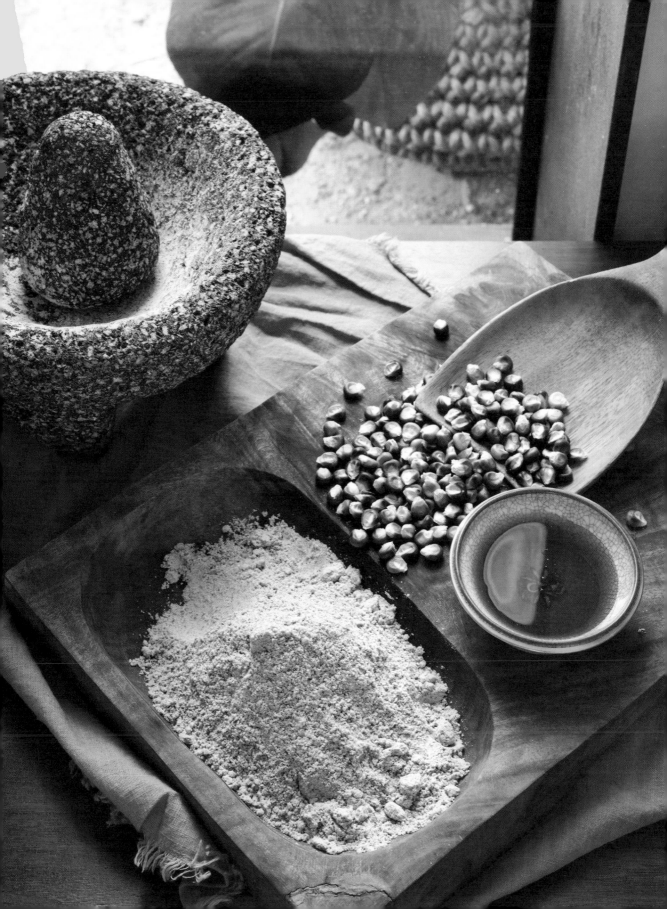

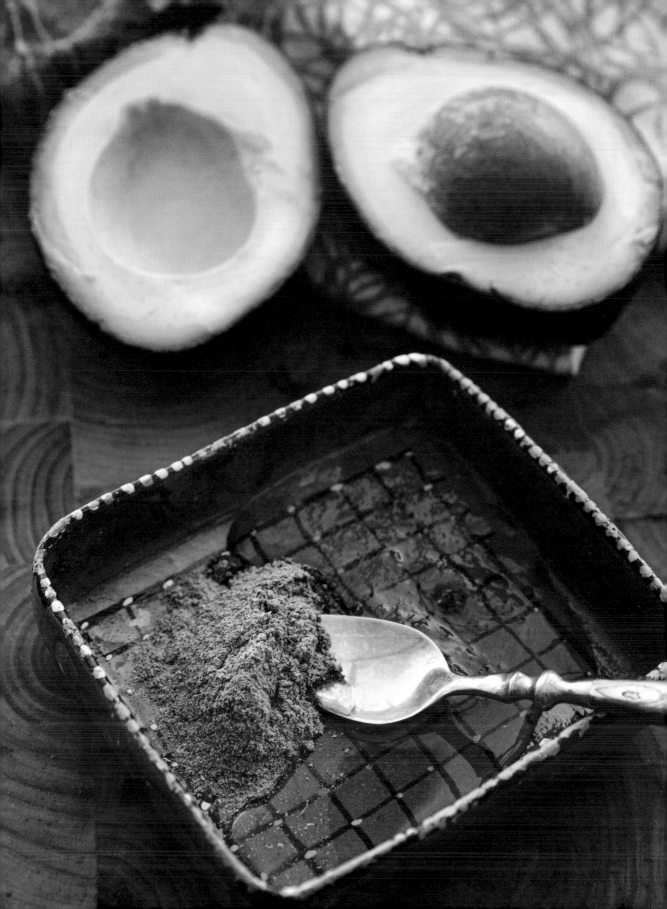

GENTLE STRENGTH FACE MASK

When I was first exploring natural body care and food, I had a favorite store I would visit in Tempe, Arizona, called Gentle Strength Co-op. It was more than a "health food" store—it was a space for those in our community who shared similar ideas and goals to meet and support one another during a time when American diets were shifting and beauty standards were far from natural. It was where I learned about the macrobiotic diet and tried wheatgrass juice.

The high oxygen content of chlorophyll in wheatgrass makes it superior in helping deliver more oxygen to our blood. Touted as a powerful detoxifier, when taken internally, wheatgrass offers over 100 elements that are essential for vital health! When applied to our skin, it can help with the effects of premature aging due to its potent antioxidants, vitamins, and minerals.

This mask not only brings a strong dose of oxygen to your face in the form of wheatgrass, but it also gently rejuvenates your skin with powerful healers using aloe vera, avocado, and honey. What a perfect name for this mask, made first with ingredients I found at Gentle Strength.

Makes 1 mask

½ small avocado, peeled
2 tablespoons aloe vera gel (see page 27)
1 teaspoon honey
1 teaspoon powdered wheatgrass

Using a fork, mash the avocado in a small bowl until smooth. Add the remaining ingredients and mix well using a small spoon. To use the mask, apply to a clean face using your fingertips and leave on the skin for 15 minutes. Rinse with warm water. Pat dry. Store any remaining mask in a glass jar in the refrigerator for up to 1 week.

BOTANICA FACE STEAM RITUAL

Botanicas are more than storefronts. They are gathering places, spaces of wonder, and suppliers of our spiritual practices. There are many types of botanicas, each serving their community with prepared remedies, spiritual supplies, and dried herbs that are unique to their tradition. In the Southwest, many of our botanicas reflect our Mexican community, whereas in other parts of the country, such as on the East Coast and in the South, you will find plenty more botanicas of African-based traditional beliefs. Regardless of the tradition, most botanicas will hit you with their scent the moment you walk in the door. Spiritual perfumes, incense, herbs, and candles all hold sacred space in a botanica. Each store holds an energy of their own, and when I find one that resonates with my spirit, I tend to make my visit a special outing for the day with a friend.

Here in the desert, where the air is very dry, my skin loves when I use my cool mist humidifier, hydrosols, and face steams with herbs from my local botanica. Although I do not have time to do this ritual every night, when I do set aside the time, I always have glowing skin the following day. Herbal steam opens your pores and helps remove impurities while the aromatics help you breathe more clearly. Look for a special candle while you're at the botanica to use while blending and setting intentions into your ingredients.

Makes 1½ cups of the herbal blend

You can easily adapt the yield of this recipe to suit your needs by measuring equal amounts of each herb.

¼ **cup dried mint**
¼ **cup dried calendula petals**
¼ **cup dried lavender buds**
¼ **cup dried rose petals**
¼ **cup dried rosemary leaves**
¼ **cup dried chamomile buds**
12-ounce glass jar

In a medium bowl, mix all the ingredients together with a spoon or your hands. Store the mixture in the glass jar with a label.

To steam your face, place one tablespoon of the herbal mixture into the large bowl. Add 3 cups of boiling water to the herbs and allow the mixture to infuse for one minute. Drape a large towel over your head and the bowl, allowing the steam to rise up onto your face. Keep your face about 6 inches away from the water and steam for 5 minutes or however long you can manage. After the water has cooled, return the water and plant material to the earth, if possible.

SPIRITUAL
WORK
WITH AIR

SACRED SCENTS INCENSE

I grew up in a culture where burning plant aromatics was part of our family's culture and used in many ceremonial events such as Pueblo Feast Days, where cedar and pine torches are burned. I have been taught that burning our ancestral aromatics takes us back to the sacred places of our ancestors and helps us remember who we are. The use of fragrant smoke as a conduit to connect with the element of Air and our ancestors is powerful.

Burning aromatics has been used in traditional healing for time immemorial, which means it should be treated respectfully. I do my best to stay educated on plants that have now become endangered and threatened from recent trends resulting in overuse. Many indigenous plants, including California white sage and Peruvian palo santo, have been overharvested and now require time to regenerate. Copal resin, the plant aromatic I work with most, is harvested from bountiful and fast-growing trees in Mexico and Central America. I use it as the base for so many of my incense recipes along with sandalwood from plantations in Australia. When choosing plant material for your own personal blends, consider including plants that you can grow and ones that are ancestral to you. Also, source out ones that are in abundance and collected ethically.

UNBOUND INCENSE

Making your own loose incense is not complicated. I like experimenting with different combinations first as a loose incense to gauge their scent combination before I make them into cones, so be sure to keep a notebook close by for your recipes. I generally use a 1:1:1 ratio of herbs, resins, and woods. You may be called to a specific plant that carries a special meaning to you. Or, you may simply be drawn to an aromatic based on their scent alone.

Amount varies

Choose one each of the following:
Herbs: anise seed, bay leaves, calendula flowers, cedar leaves, cloves, fennel seeds, fir needles, gingerroot, juniper berries, lavender flowers, mugwort, orange peel, rose petals, rosemary, star anise, sweetgrass
Resin (small pieces or powdered): benzoin, copal, dragon's blood, myrrh, piñon
Woods: birch, cinnamon bark, cedarwood, juniper, piñon, sandalwood

Incense burning vessel
Earth (salt, sand, or dirt)
Bamboo charcoal tablets for incense burning
Matches

Choose your 3 plant materials, one each of herbs, resin, and woods. Working in small batches is best, so only use a teaspoon or tablespoon of each and place into a small bowl. Mix with a spoon.

To burn your incense, place the earth you chose at the bottom of your incense burning vessel. Next, place a bamboo charcoal tablet on top of the earth. Using a match, light your tablet and wait for sparks to work through the charcoal. Place a pinch of your mixture on top of the tablet, allowing it to permeate the air.

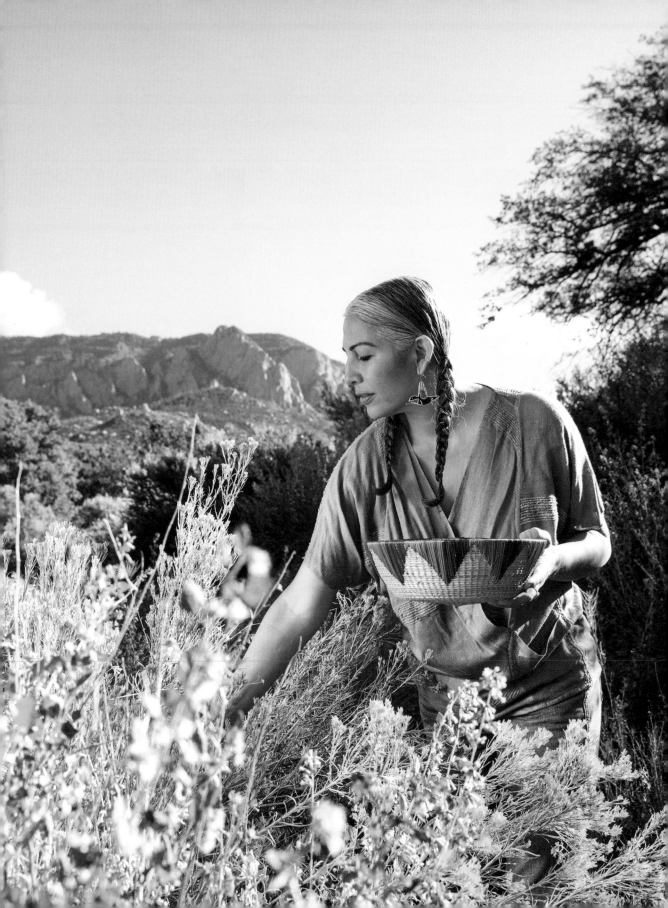

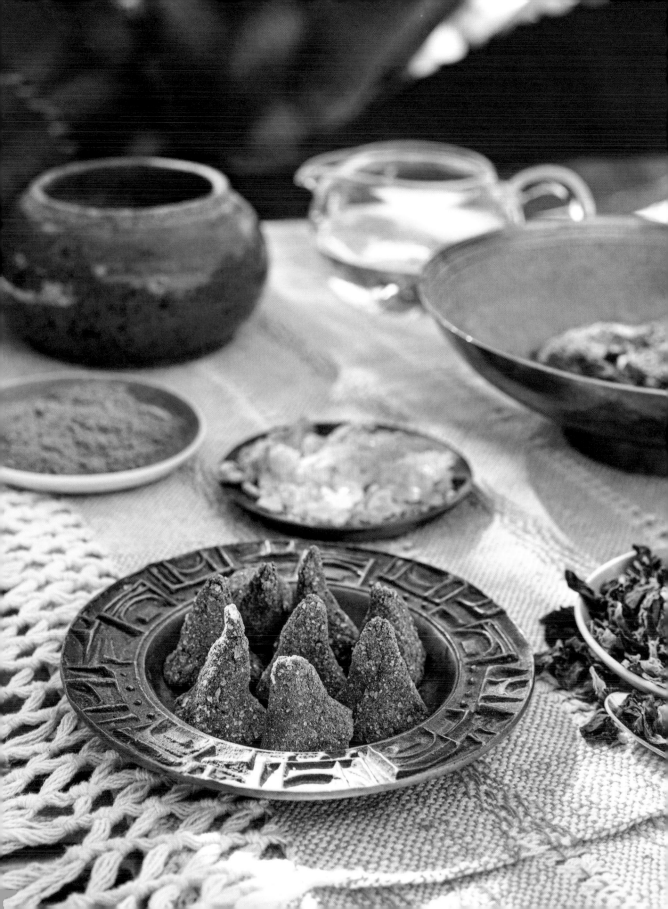

LA GUADALUPANA CONES

This incense blend came to me in a dream long ago. Our Lady of Guadalupe, also known as Earth Mother Tonantzin, has a complicated history and is known to many as *Mother to the People of Mexico*. She has become a symbol of hope and love to many Indigenous peoples, including my own Mexican community. La Guadalupana's flower is said to be the rose, the flower which carries the highest frequency on our planet. When combined with copal, sandalwood, and cinnamon, the sweet scent not only invokes the element of Air but her warm embrace as well.

Amount varies

Making cone incense can be a bit of trial and error until you get your ratios just right. I suggest you start small, beginning with one teaspoon for each part.

2 parts finely ground Mexican copal resin

2 parts sandalwood powder

1 part ground cinnamon

1 part ground rose petals

1 part makko powder

About 4 parts water

Dropper

Measure out the dried ingredients and add to a small bowl. Combine with a spoon. Next, add a tiny amount of water using your dropper and stir with a spoon. If you add too much water the mixture will be sticky and won't form into cones, so it is best to start with a small amount.

Mix the blend until you have a pliable dough. If it is crumbling, you need to add a few more drops of water. Knead it with your fingers until you have a slightly tacky dough, then pinch off pieces

(continued)

and shape them into cones. Place them on a plate or tray to dry. The drying time will vary depending on the time of year and humidity. Here in the desert, my cones take just one day to dry in the sun.

To burn your incense, place one cone on a heat-resistant surface and light the top. Sometimes cones will not burn the whole way through depending on the plants used. If this happens, simply put your cone on a charcoal tablet as you would with loose incense.

SKY NATION VISITS

Artemisia ludoviciana, Grandmother Sage, western mugwort, or iztauhyatl and estafiate as I was taught, is native throughout the entire Western United States and south into Mexico. It is one of the most popular plants used in Mexican herbalism and its applications are many. It can be made into a tea for chest congestion or a poultice for insect bites, used for moxibustion during pregnancy, or its aromatic smoke can be utilized as a remedy for *mal aire*—which is said to be associated with headaches or sudden fright.

Traditionally, it is also used for dreaming. Since I was thirteen, I have been receiving messages from spirits during my dreamtime, so this is my favorite way to honor this plant. Dreams are associated with the element of Air as they are a form of communication, knowledge, and inspiration. These visits from the Sky Nation come unexpectedly, presenting clear information for me and, more often, for others. Sharing these messages with people over the past three decades has been a gift and sometimes a hardship. However, I always welcome them lovingly as the messenger and believer of psychic faculties. I work with estafiate as well as another Mexican herb called calea zacatechichi to encourage visits from the Sky Nation People and to help recall their messages. I have only been able to find this bitter herb while in Mexico or online in specialty herbal stores. If you cannot find it dried for the following recipe, try looking for it as an herbal tincture to add to hot water.

As with everything, intention is vital. When you work with estafiate, be crystal clear by stating your intention and asking her kindly to help bring you sweet dreams and clarity and to remember your dreams upon waking.

SKY NATION TEA

Makes 2 servings

1 tablespoon calea zacatechichi
2 cups water
Natural sweetener (honey or maple syrup)

Bring the water to a boil in a small saucepan fitted with a lid. Turn off the heat, add the calea zacatechichi, and cover the pot, allowing the herb to infuse for about 20 minutes. Strain and add a sweetener to taste if you'd like.

For the ritual, set your intention for the tea and sip on a cup of the beverage about 30 minutes to 1 hour before bedtime, being mindful that drinking too much tea will cause you to wake to use the restroom.

SKY NATION SACHETS

1 part dried estafiate leaves
1 part dried lavender flowers
Muslin bags, any size of your preference

Mix your herbs in a small bowl and fill your sachet using a spoon.

For the ritual, set your intention while deeply breathing in your sachet before placing it in your pillowcase for the evening. Have a dream journal nearby.

(continued)

SKY NATION INCENSE

Heatproof vessel to burn your incense
Earth (sand or dirt)
Charcoal tablets for incense
Loose, dried estafiate

To induce dreams, this incense is best burned in the evening. Place your incense burner on a heat-resistant surface and put a few spoons of the earth you chose on the bottom of the burner. Place your charcoal tablet on the earth and light. Once it is hot, place a small pinch of estafiate on top of the charcoal and allow it to burn in a well-ventilated area.

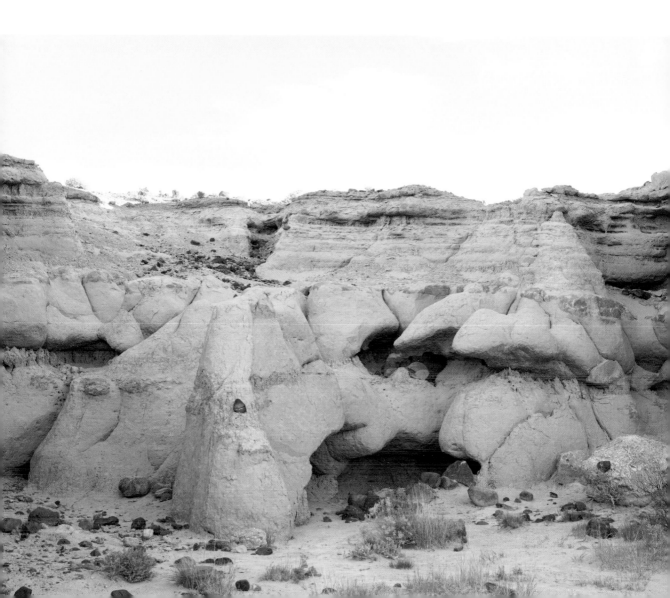

PLUMED SERPENT
BREATHING EXERCISE

Many years ago, on a trip to the highlands of Mexico, I had the opportunity to visit the pyramid of Xochicalco. Its name, meaning "Hill of Flowers" in Nahuatl, is the site to a ceremonial center, ancient ball courts, and other pyramids including the Pyramid of the Plumed Serpent. The Pyramid of the Plumed Serpent is covered in beautiful bas-relief carvings, including the symbol of Quetzalcoatl in the image of Ehécatl, who represents the wind—The Plumed Serpent (see page 70). The pyramid, which is not very tall, is easy to climb and offers a rooftop view where you can take in the surrounding land.

I will never forget the day I stood on top of that pyramid. When I reached its platform, I took in a deep breath and closed my eyes. I was going through many personal trials at that time and being up there felt so serene. Eyes still closed, I felt a small gust of wind and then felt as though a beam of light had entered the top of my head. With the wind came a message. I remember opening my eyes, feeling totally at peace and full of insight. I knew exactly what I had to do next regarding some very difficult life decisions.

That day, with all its magic, was one of the most powerful experiences of my adult life. When I feel I need to channel a deeper intuition, I imagine myself back on top of that pyramid with the Plumed Serpent and I focus on my breathing. Air is the element of inspiration, knowledge, learning, and intuition. So, when you are feeling stuck or know you are ready for change, look to Air for guidance. I have now incorporated this simple breathing exercise into my own private practice, and I guide others using the image of this beautiful serpent.

(continued)

Sitting comfortably in a quiet space, relax and breathe with your natural rhythm. Using your mind's eye, imagine a beautiful feathered serpent moving through the air in a playful zigzag fashion. Now, envision the serpent flying gently around your body, creating wind with its movement. It's creating energy that is guiding you into motion. Inhale and exhale using your natural breath. Now in your mind's eye, imagine a beam of light entering the crown of your head. Focus on this light and all the cosmic energy it brings to you. Continue breathing in your natural breath. Trust your intuition and listen to what the light is telling you. The serpent now flies away, and the light retracts back up to the sky. Sit quietly, breathing your natural breath. Release any constructs you may be holding on to and focus on your awakened perception. Open your eyes when you are ready.

Icaros of the Wind

When gathering plants or making my plant remedies I oftentimes find myself humming or singing. It is something that I have done since I was a young girl, and I believe it was passed down from my Aunt Helen on my father's side. As I grew older and began studying and learning various curanderismo traditions, one modality that resonated with my heart was the use of *icaros*. Performing icaros is used by many curanderas, mostly of South American traditions, as a ritual act. Using gentle singing, chants, humming, or melodic whistling, icaros help to invest a person or plant with protection and healing energy.

Sound has been used as a spiritual tool by various cultures for thousands of years, and in my own practice, I include sound healing with icaros—my drum, rattle, and bells—to establish and restore harmony within my own body and the energies of my clients. However, any sound can be used as a healing tool if the intention of the instrument being played is used to bring about balance. Wind chimes are Mother Earth's instrument, as they capture the element of Air and create their own personal icaros for us to hear. Made from various materials such as shells, metal, or wood, wind chimes sing songs of peace and awareness and protect us from evil forces with their tones and heavenly frequencies.

I encourage my students and clients to invest in a wind chime for their spaces as I believe it's a wonderful tool to bring in peace with the element of Air. My favorite wind chimes are made of metal, but it's important to choose a wind chime that resonates with you and sings your tune.

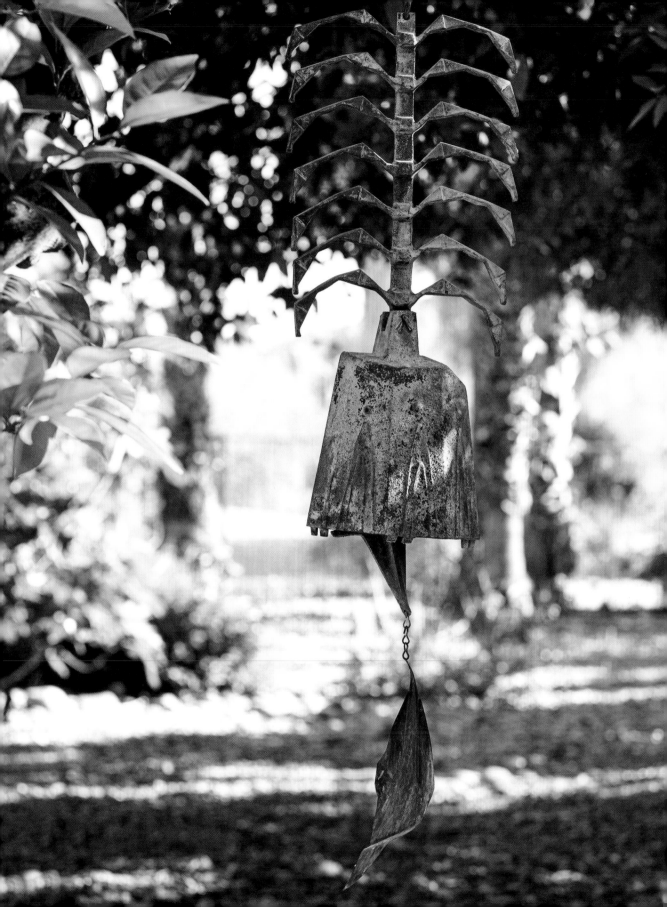

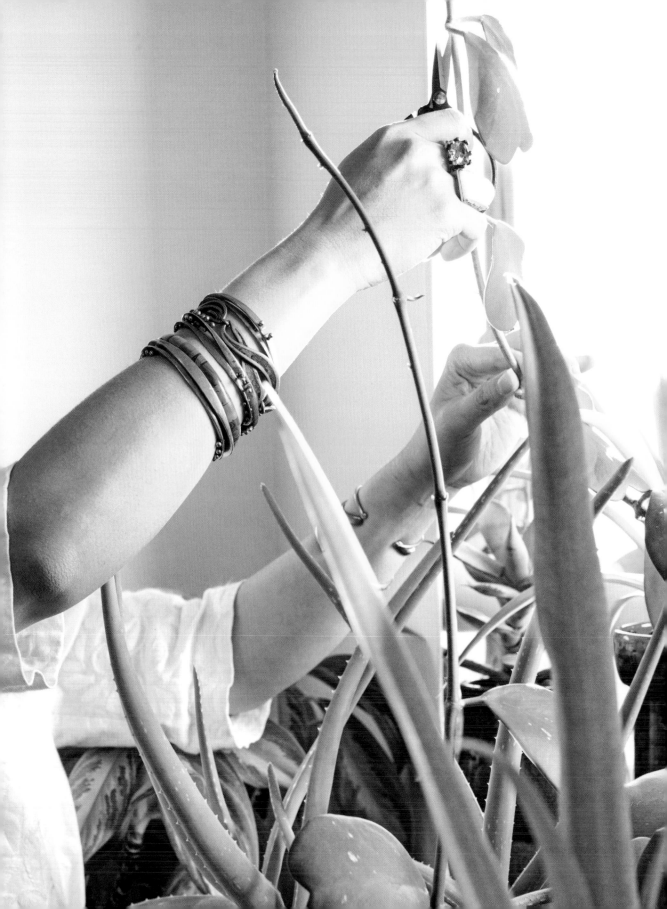

HOUSEPLANTS

Often, our indoor air can be more polluted than outdoor air. Using plants for purification in your home can help in removing indoor pollutants while improving the quality of air. A few of my houseplants have been rescued from the side of the street and others were adopted from friends who were moving. I love talking to them, watching them sprout new growth, and when I leave for vacation, I worry about them as though I were leaving a pet. I nurture them just as much as they nurture me, and oftentimes, I find myself sharing plant babies with friends to propagate their unfolding beauty.

Plants, like people, come in different shapes, sizes, and have their own unique personalities. So, whether you desire to make a bold statement with a big-leafed tropical plant or are more interested in something low-maintenance, all plants will add texture and interest to your home. Growing fresh air is fun, and the more plants you have, the more they can do for the Air quality of the space you inhabit. Keeping houseplants allows us to have little healing filters right in our own homes.

Commitment: Like pets, houseplants need to be taken care of. Tropical varieties may need a misting of water to keep them happy, while others, such as succulents, are low-maintenance, only needing water now and then. Visit your local nursery and ask which plant best suits your level of commitment.

Indoor Light: Assess your living space to determine which plants will do best in your environment. All houseplants need sunlight to thrive; however, some will do fine with less natural light than others. Most houseplants will enjoy eastern- and western-facing windows.

Toxic Plants: Some plants are toxic if eaten or touched by little ones or pets. So, take some basic safety measures and read up on which plants are best for your children or pets.

THE SPEAKING FEATHER

The winged ones, such as hawks, hummingbirds, and quetzales, teach us about perspective and liberation. Since I was a little girl, I have especially loved birds—so much so that I named my daughter *Paloma*, which means "dove" in Spanish. The dove, symbolizing peace worldwide, holds attributes I desired for her in hopes she would experience peace as she grew into her being. *Having inner peace allows one to create peace.* And like most birds, doves demonstrate freedom through their gift of flight. The ability to glide through air and see from another perspective reminds us how to be visionaries, better communicators, and empaths.

Before my speaking engagements, I take a moment to gain clarity so that I may communicate effectively. In my mind's eye, I envision myself flying about the room observing the audience with keen vision. I see their body language, the clothes that they're wearing, who they are with, their age, and so on. It's a mindfulness tool I use to sense the energy around the room, as speaking in front of people used to bring me great anxiety. Now I keep a feather in my notes to remind myself to fly beforehand, calling it my Speaking Feather.

Find or purchase a feather, any size or color, that speaks to you. Before speaking in front of a group, hold your feather and say to yourself:

Winged Ones, help me gain a wider perspective. Let me see with absolute clarity. Help me speak my truth and rise above even Myself.

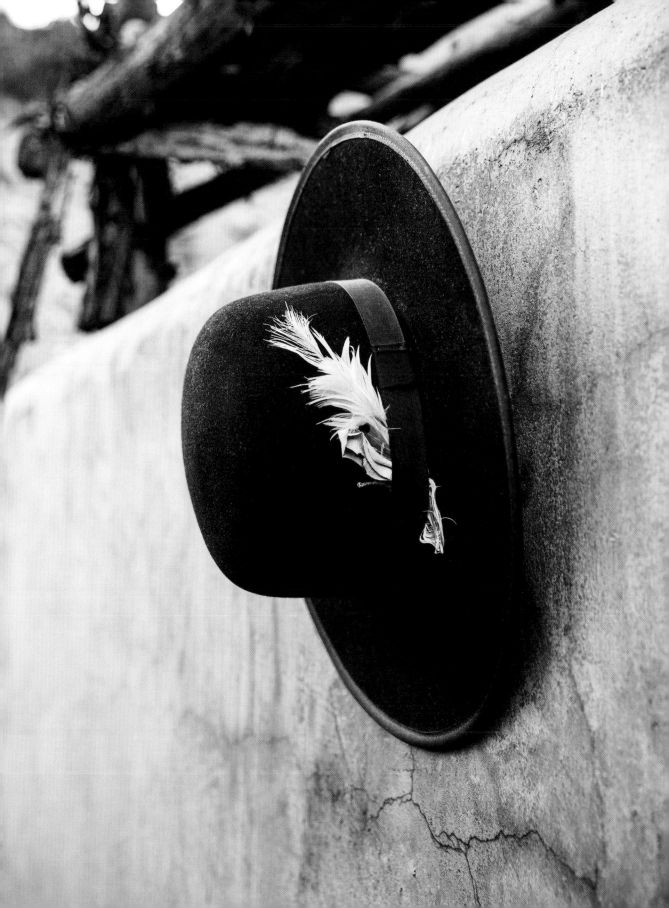

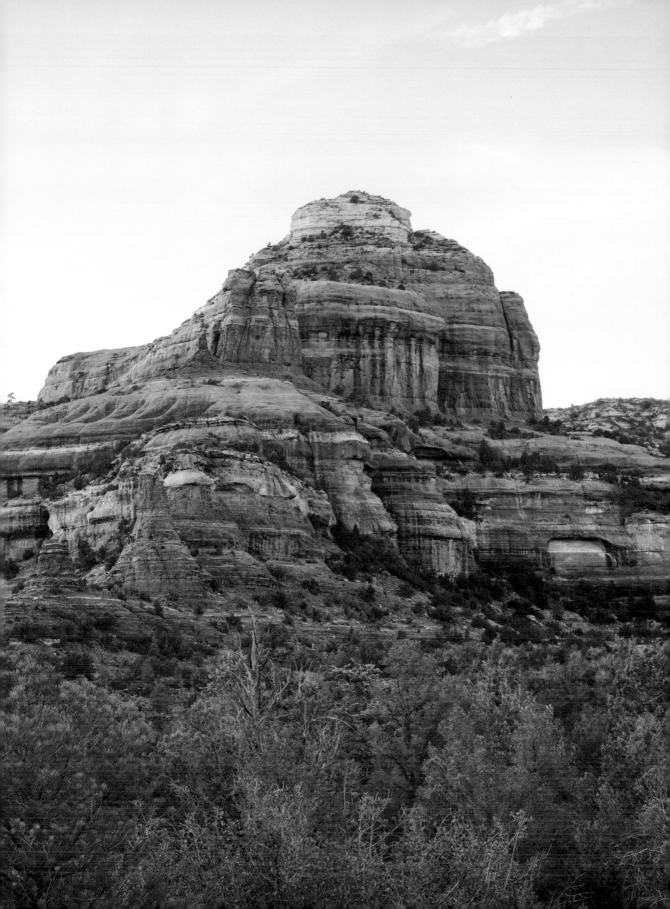

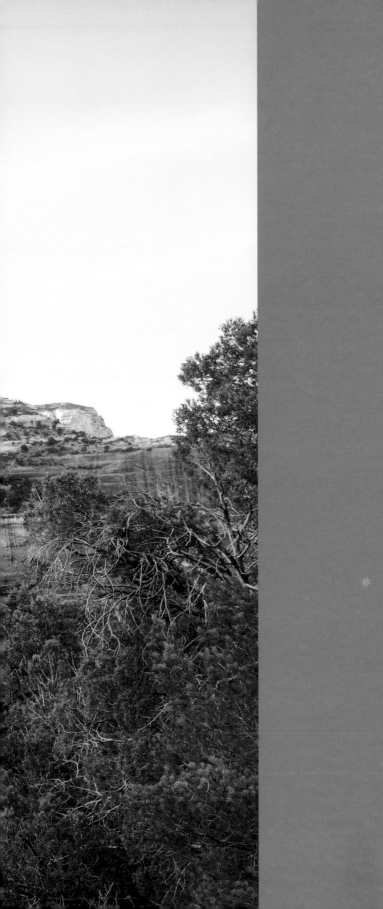

111 ◇ EARTH

PRAYER TO EARTH

Nourishing, grounding, and precious Earth, you are the wise Mother to all that lives upon your back. Your unconditional love supports me and keeps me rooted. When I feel disharmony, your constant guidance can be sensed by simply standing on your being. I honor and thank you for allowing me to embody your spirit through your Earth medicines and ask you to forgive us humans for not caring for you as we should. May we see ourselves in every living being, and may we heal you as you continue to heal us.

EARTH FOR INNER HARMONY

THE BEAUTY OF EARTH

SPIRITUAL WORK WITH EARTH

EARTH IS THE COLLECTVE HOME FOR ALL LIFE:

living waters, breathing forests, and the planetary citizens composed of her earthly elements. Mother Earth, Pachamama, Madre Tierra— whichever name you choose to use, now more than ever we must act as a collective and call on her name to listen to her sacred teachings. In many of my Indigenous talking circles, there is much discussion on the healing and protection of Mother Earth. From the water protectors who organized at Standing Rock in 2016 to the plant allies speaking on behalf of our plants on the verge of extinction, people are coming together across the globe to defend our Mother's gifts. However, Earth's vast offerings are not simply limited to her natural resources. Life lessons are also found deep within her seasons, natural design, environments, and history.

Earth wisdom teaches us about cycles, reciprocity, empathy, renewal, equilibrium, wholeness, roots, and foresight. When we put into place these lessons and teachings, we feel centered, grounded, secure, and supported. This can be achieved by eating seasonal foods, hiking in the mountains, using only what we need, or simply saying thank you to the ancestors who lived under different circumstances. The Earth element is like the cement platform of a new home. It provides a solid base on which to build, and we too need a strong foundation to expand and thrive. This foundation of our health and well-being is shaped in part by how we respond to internal and external conditions. Thankfully, Earth supplies us with all we need for a healthy inner body through the abundance of plants and minerals found in her soil and waters. However, our modern lifestyles have pulled us away from Earth, leaving many of us in less than optimal health.

Throughout my life, many have contacted me for herbal suggestions to help heal their bodies with no desire to make external adjustments to their lifestyle. This magic-pill mentality will not heal us collectively; that mindset places power on the herbs and not on the person themselves. We are all healers, and our healing arises from within, supported by Earth's bounty of medicines.

One of my favorite ways of incorporating Earth's bounty into my daily life is by indulging in her natural ingredients. Many world beauty practices use Earth's ingredients not only for beauty regimens but also in ritual to celebrate one's marriage or pregnancy. I love creating simple products for my own personal use as well as sharing ways in which others can treat their skin to a daily ritual to keep it soft and supple. However, beauty is only skin deep—while someone may appear beautiful on the outside, their character isn't necessarily beautiful on the inside. This also holds true for many commercial beauty products whose gorgeous packaging are filled with harsh chemicals and synthetic ingredients. Consider this is a reminder that true beauty is first being comfortable in your own packaging, and then honoring it with Earth's ingredients for cleansing, hydration, and defense.

As I write this entry for the Earth chapter, I cannot help but reflect on the time that I am writing these words, spring 2020. In many Native American teachings, spring is represented by the Earth element, symbolizing an awakening that brings forth new energy in one's life and in the Earth itself. Now in the depths of the COVID-19 pandemic this spring, I find myself thinking often about the Earth element and praying for blessings of renewal and stability for my family, friends, and community on our Earth walk. The spirit of Nature gives us the ability to spiritually go deep within ourselves once we recognize we *are* a part of Nature. Because we have gradually disconnected from her source of energy over the past few decades, I believe this is why we are intuitively being called back at this time to reconnect with her organic matter.

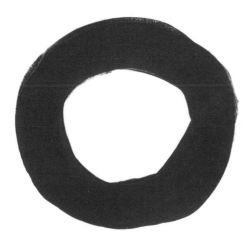

EARTH
FOR INNER
HARMONY

YERBA BUENA
CACAO BITES

Home remedies are very important in many Mexican American households from the use of simple infusions such as *manzanilla* (chamomile) for calming nerves to yerba buena (spearmint) for an upset stomach. And although these two herbs were introduced by the Spanish, our abuelitas have long incorporated them into our healing traditions with yerba buena being one of the most widely used herbs found in many homes. Yerba buena, which means "good herb" in Spanish, is most often used fresh. There are several varieties of mints that grow wild depending on where you live; however, many of the grandmothers I learned from here in the Southwest and California all had common spearmint growing in abundance by their front doors or in their backyards. In some homes where grandmas had an abundance of yerba buena, they would even make little bundles to hang by an open window so they could catch a breeze, releasing their scent to purify and sweeten the room.

The Earth element is associated with abundance, nourishment, and all good things in life—bringing the words "the sweet life" to mind. When I work with fresh yerba buena, I instantly have thoughts of this sweet life with its scent of kindness and taste of nourishing medicine. I never grow immune to its fragrance, and I love watching how people react when they breathe it in. We can all use a reminder now and then about how sweet life really is. Take a moment to reflect on all the abundance and nourishment the Earth provides for us. These little cacao bites are very easy to create, and I like doubling the recipe to share with friends or give to my clients as a treat after their sessions.

(continued)

1 cup raw cacao butter

1 cup raw cacao powder

2 tablespoons fresh spearmint, minced, or 1 tablespoon dried

½ cup raw honey

Sea salt

Silicone molds in your desired shape and size (I use two 1-by-1-inch molds)

Using a double boiler (see page 12), melt the cacao butter. When it's melted, add the cacao powder and stir until smooth. Next, add the spearmint, honey, and a pinch of sea salt, and mix well. Pour or spoon the mixture into the silicone molds and refrigerate at least 1 hour. Remove the bites from the molds and store them in the refrigerator or freezer.

Abuelita's Yerba Buena Tea: For Colds, Headaches, and Stomachaches

Gather a small handful of fresh yerba buena. Rinse and place the leaves and stems in a large mug. Pour boiling water over them, cover, and infuse for at least 10 minutes. Depending on your preference, you can remove the herbs or keep them in the mug and eat them afterward. Add honey to taste if desired.

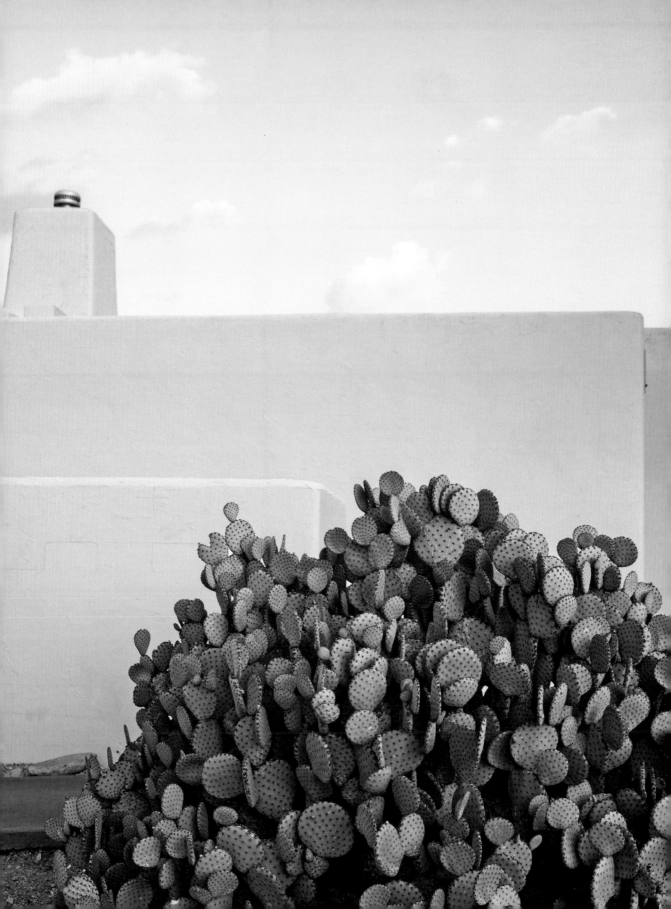

ROOT MEDICINE FOR IMMUNE SUPPORT

This recipe is taken from a workshop I taught on incorporating indigenous plants into your kitchen medicine. The students loved it because it was a simple home remedy using dried and fresh roots, and it felt very witchy with all the constant stirring of ingredients in the double boiler.

Echinacea purpurea is an incredible herb for immune support and has long been used as medicine by Indigenous tribes of North America for countless generations, including the Kiowa and Sioux. I like mentioning little facts like these because I find that students believe echinacea to be native to Europe since it is often marketed as such. Many of the plants we use in today's folk medicine–making were first used as medicine by the Indigenous peoples of the Americas long before they traveled to Europe.

This recipe includes *sauco*, which is Mexican elderflower. If you cannot find Mexican elderflower, which grows all over the Southwest, you can easily substitute European elderflower with the same results.

Makes about 1 cup

1 cup honey

1 tablespoon dried sauco (Mexican elderflower)

2 tablespoons fresh gingerroot, diced

2 tablespoons fresh horseradish root, diced

1 tablespoon dried echinacea root

8-ounce glass jar

Boil water in the bottom of a double boiler (see page 12). Add raw honey in the top pan of the double boiler. Next, add the sauco, gingerroot, horseradish root, and echinacea root to the honey and stir well. Heat your mixture over very low heat, stirring occasionally, for at least 1 hour. Do not allow the mixture to rise above 110 degrees—you can use a food thermometer to keep an eye on this. After the herbs have infused, allow the elixir to cool slightly. Pour it through a fine mesh strainer into a clean, dry jar and label it.

To use this root medicine, enjoy a spoonful for daily immune support or use it in your favorite herbal tea during times of cold and flu.

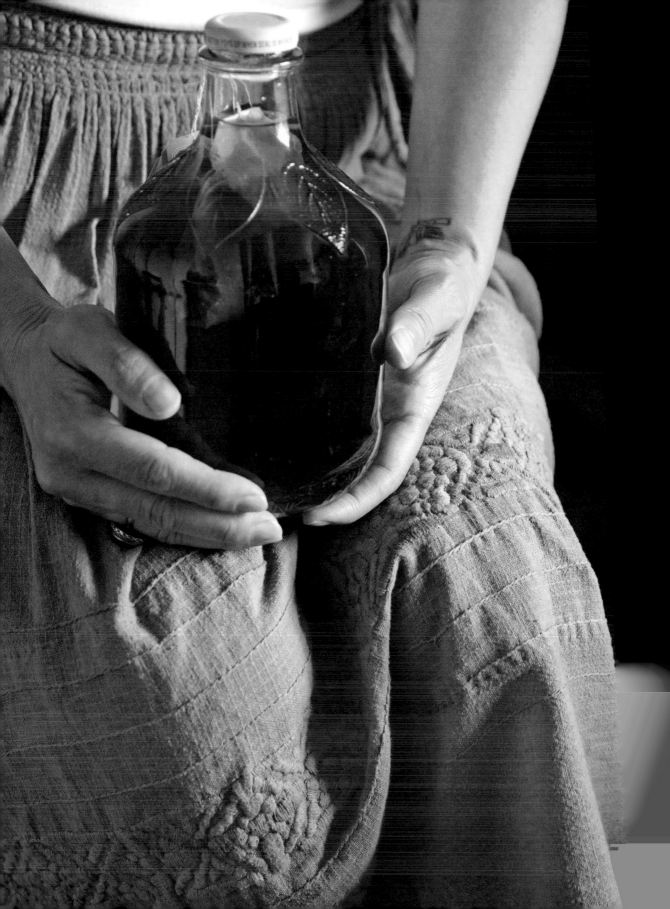

MAYAN TEA TO CALM THE MIND

Poch'il is the Mayan word for "passionflower" (*Passiflora incarnata*), which is a gorgeous climbing vine that grows throughout the Americas. As a child, my family had one of the many hundreds of species of poch'il climbing on a trellis on our front porch. I loved looking into the purple flowers with a magnifying glass and seeing all the complex little parts inside. It is such a strange flower with an even stranger (to me) history that had nothing to do with passion as I know it today.

When Spaniards were colonizing the Americas in the sixteenth century, they learned about the plant from the Indigenous peoples of the area who used it in their bush medicines, which included various flowers, barks, and roots. And although it went by many traditional names, it was soon renamed passionflower by the Spaniards because it resembles the crown of thorns. "The Passion" is a term used in Christianity to describe the final period of Jesus's life when he wore a crown of thorns.

Along with the poch'il, I've included lemongrass and spearmint in this tea blend. These are two common herbs used by modern-day Mayans and Garifunas who continue to practice bush medicine by incorporating traditional and faraway plants that have been adopted into their apothecary. Lemongrass is speculated to be native to Southern India, Sri Lanka, or Malaysia, and spearmint is native to Europe and Asia. Like poch'il, both are good for calming the stomach and mind.

(continued)

Makes about 1 cup

½ cup dried poch'il
¼ cup dried lemongrass
¼ cup dried spearmint
8-ounce glass jar

Measure out the herbs, mix them together, and put them in the glass jar. Seal the jar and label it.

To make the tea, use 1 teaspoon of the blend per each cup (about 8 ounces) of water. Bring the water to a boil in a small saucepan or teakettle. Place your desired amount of the herbal mixture in a tea infuser, tea bag, or French press. Pour boiling water over the herbs and infuse for 5 to 7 minutes. Strain and enjoy.

ZARZAPARRILLA
ADAPTOGENIC TONIC

After the Spanish arrived in Central Mexico, ranches were eventually established and stocked with cattle from Spain. By the 1700s, cattle ranching had reached far to the north, in what is now Arizona, New Mexico, and Texas, bringing horses and Indigenous Mexicans and their medicines. Roots such as zarzaparrilla were gathered by Native people yearlong, dried in the sun, and then tied in bundles to be sold locally for medicine or exported to the north, where the curanderas would include them in their tonics. And although the *vaqueros* (cowboys) of the time were drinking zarzaparrilla mainly as a remedy for syphilis, this root medicine goes back much further than that.

Zarzaparrilla (*Smilax ornata*) is a prickly vine that is native to Southern Mexico, the Caribbean, and Central and South America and is used by Indigenous peoples for numerous ailments. It roughly translates as "brambly little vine" and also goes by sarsaparilla. All parts of the plant are used as medicine, with their thin roots being used most notably in old-fashioned root beer.

As a descendant of vaqueros, ranch workers, nurses, and folk healers, I imagine a tonic such as this would have been given as a treatment for many conditions. I envision long-ago grandmas preparing it as a tea or spring tonic and adding it to coffee to help with the stressors of the time. Zarzaparrilla has been shown to be a great adaptogen, meaning it helps the body adapt to stressful conditions. Personally, I like to drink a mug of the root when I am in the middle of a big project and need a little grounding. Traditionally, this tonic would be made simply with water, but I love the way it tastes when paired with a creamy nondairy milk such as hemp milk. I think my ancestors would approve.

Makes 1 serving

1 cup nondairy milk
1 teaspoon ground or finely chopped zarzaparrilla root
Pinch of cayenne
Honey

In a small saucepan, bring the milk to almost-boiling. Turn the temperature down to a simmer. Add the zarzaparrilla root and cayenne to the milk and simmer for 5 minutes. Pour into a mug. Sweeten with honey and enjoy.

LA ARCILLA
GENTLE CLEANSE

When I was pregnant with my daughter, I had a strong urge to taste dirt. I would wet my index finger with saliva and touch the ground in my backyard to pick up a few traces of soil to taste in my mouth. It was so satisfying, and yet I was so embarrassed to tell anyone about this odd craving. It would be years later that I would read research on this very topic, pregnant women craving earth.

Arcilla or "wet earth," has been used traditionally in many cultures for its healing properties, including removing toxins. Some rural Peruvian farmers even make a sauce that includes clay to serve alongside wild potatoes. The practice of ingesting clay for stomach ailments has been well-researched in present and ancient cultures spanning the world. One example is from Indigenous peoples of the Southwest, where clay is baked with acorn flour to reduce the toxicity of the acorns.

For a gentle cleanse, I drink a small amount of clay that is labeled safe for internal use (such as most bentonite clays), dissolved in water to help with my digestion when it feels sluggish. This is not something I do often, but when I drink it, it always tastes good to me.

Makes 1 serving

½ **teaspoon bentonite clay**
½ **cup to 1 cup water**

Add your clay and desired amount of water to a glass, stir. Drink straightaway or allow the clay to settle and simply drink the cloudy water.

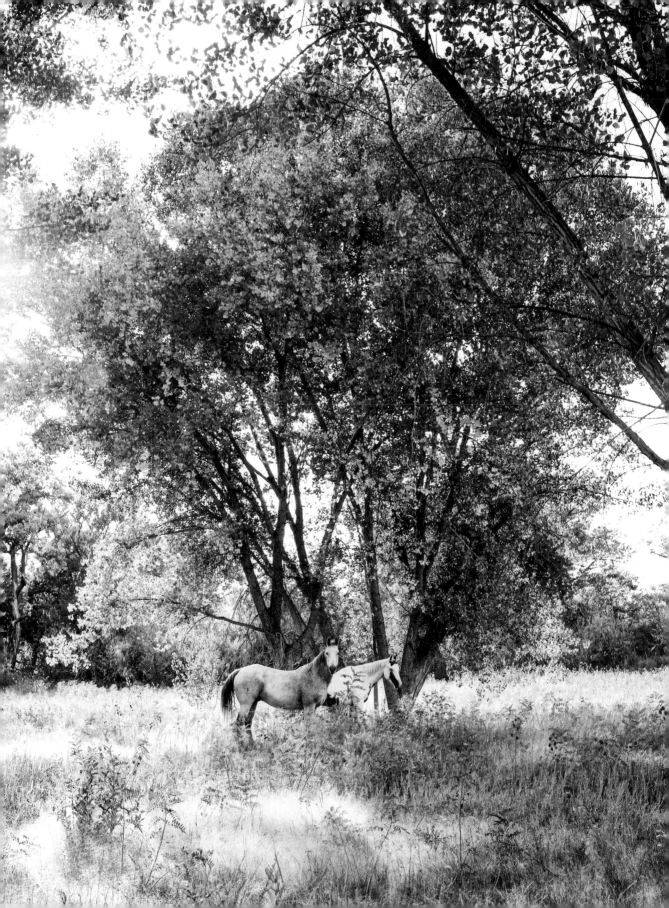

THE BEAUTY OF EARTH

ROOT CHAKRA LIP TINT

The root chakra governs your inner sense of security and place on Earth. Located at the base of your spine, the root chakra, when overactive, can trigger extreme feelings of insecurity; however, when balanced, you feel present, confident, and capable. The color associated with this chakra is red. Deep, earthy red represents your ancestors, vital energy, desire, passion, and power. When you are wearing red, surrounded by it in small doses, or simply imagining it in your mind's eye, it affects your stability by supporting your foundation at its core.

Wearing actual roots on your lips is a playful way to nurture your root chakra. This lip tint, made with beetroot, is symbolic of groundedness and digging deep within. It is designed to be used in conjunction with the following affirmations: *I am present. I am safe. I am at peace. I am confident. I am one.*

Makes about ¼ cup

2 tablespoons solid coconut oil

½ teaspoon beeswax pellets

1 teaspoon sweet almond oil

1 teaspoon beetroot powder

2 drops rose essential oil (optional)

Salve tins or small glass jar

For a darker tint, infuse longer. This will create a bolder color for your lips.

Using a double boiler (see page 12), melt the coconut oil and beeswax at a low temperature. Once they're melted, stir in the sweet almond oil and beetroot powder. Allow the mixture to infuse at a very low temperature for 2 hours. Remove the boiler from heat, add the rose oil, if using, and mix. Using cheesecloth or a fine mesh strainer, strain the beet mixture into a glass measuring cup and then quickly pour the mixture into your salve tins or small jar. Allow the tint to cool and use just as you would a lip balm.

DESERT HAIR WASH

I love visiting Moroccan souks and medinas. The spices, cooking tools, textiles, and natural beauty products all resonate deeply with my spirit. Among the many little things available at these markets is mineral-rich clay called *rhassoul*. Rhassoul clay comes from the Atlas Mountains in Eastern Morocco and has been used for hundreds of years for its detoxifying and nourishing properties for the hair and skin. It is considered one of the purer and rarer clays of the earth and literally means "that which washes" in Arabic.

Rhassoul clay leaves your hair shiny and soft and it can be used to cleanse and condition your hair as often as you would use commercial products. If your hair likes extra conditioning like mine sometimes does, simply add a little more jojoba oil to your recipe. To create the wash, I like to use a small wooden bowl, as I shy away from having glass in the shower. I was also taught that you should only mix clay in ceramic, glass, or wooden containers and only use nonmetal spoons to blend with.

Makes about ¼ cup

¼ cup rhassoul clay
1 tablespoon aloe vera juice
1 teaspoon jojoba oil
About 1 tablespoon orange blossom water or rose water

Place the clay, aloe vera juice, and jojoba oil in a small wooden bowl. Mix using a small wooden spoon. Add in the floral water slowly, using enough to make a paste to your desired consistency. To use the clay, dampen your hair and massage the mixture into your scalp and through your hair, all the way to your ends. Leave on your hair for 3 to 5 minutes. Rinse well.

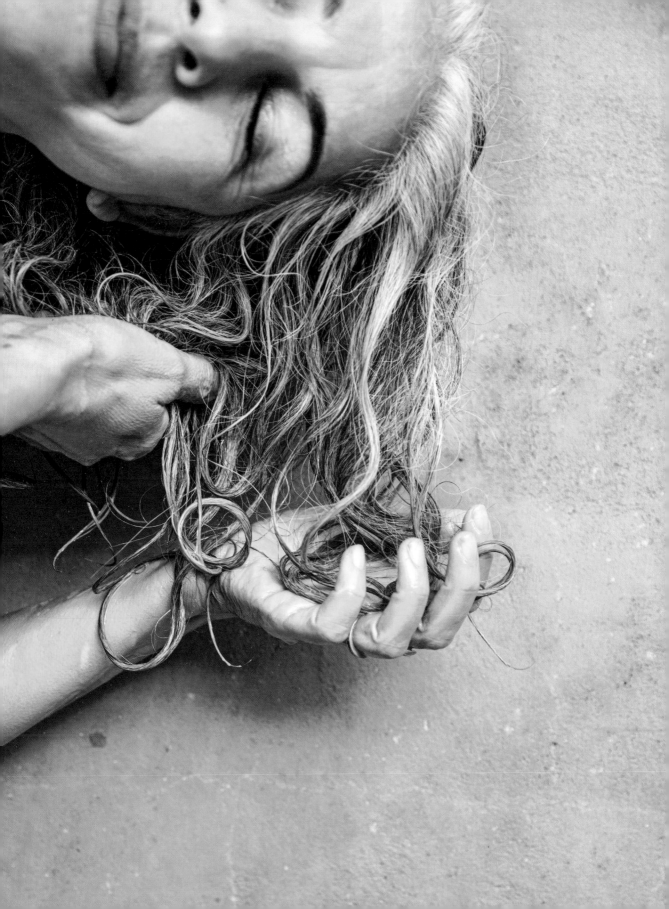

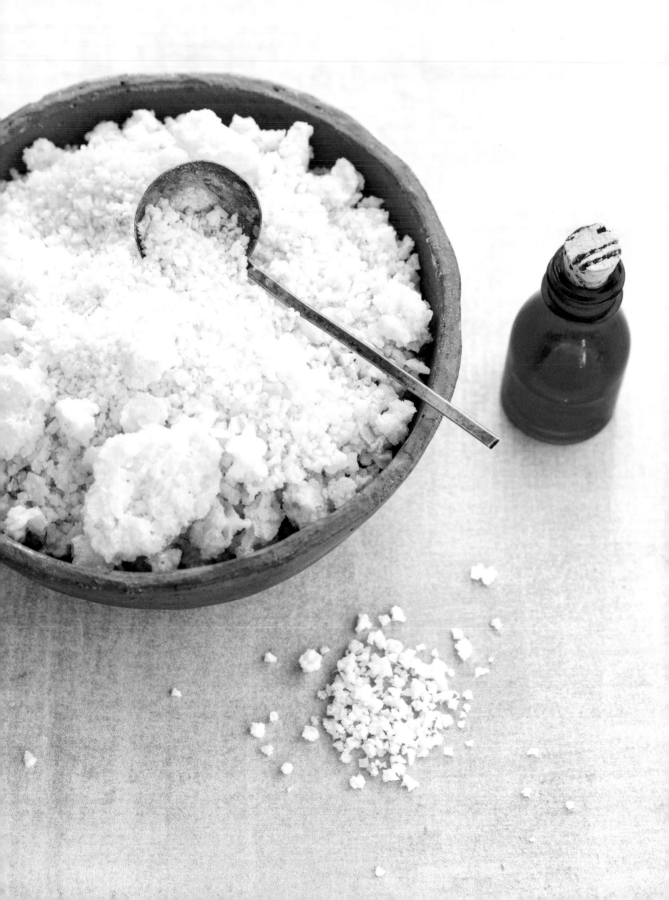

SALT OF THE EARTH DEODORANT

Salt has been an integral part of healing, commerce, and religious practices reaching all cultures across Earth since the beginning of time. Mined from caves, collected from oceans, and—in my own Pueblo traditions—harvested from Earth, salt is an incredible crystal with antimicrobial properties. When applied to our underarms, it allows us to release toxins through our sweat without all the harsh chemicals and fragrances of commercial deodorant that simply mask odor.

When I was playing with the recipe, I tried various mineral salts and found that they all worked relatively the same. The only ones I didn't try were black salts because I was afraid they would stain my clothes. In addition, I did my best to only use salts that are sustainably harvested. Due to recent trends, salts such as pink Himalayan salt are being extensively mined and will be depleted if we continue using them at the rate we are now.

For this recipe, have fun connecting to your own lineage by using salts that are related to you. For example, if you carry Greek blood, you can try a Greek sea salt to connect to Amphitrite, the Greek goddess of salt.

Makes 1 roller deodorant

2 tablespoons filtered water

1 teaspoon baking soda

1 teaspoon mineral salt, ground very fine

2 tablespoons witch hazel extract

5 drops geranium essential oil

Deodorant roller bottle, recycled or new

(continued)

In the smallest saucepan you have, bring the water to a boil. Remove it from the heat and immediately add the baking soda and salt, stirring until they have dissolved. Let the mixture cool. Meanwhile, add the witch hazel extract and essential oil to your deodorant bottle. Then, add the cooled salt solution. Place the rollerball and lid on the bottle and label it.

To use your deodorant, shake it before each use and roll a few times to apply to your underarm area, repeating later in the day as needed.

MOROCCAN SHAVING JELLY

One of the many things that caught my attention when I visited Morocco were the street shavers. These barbers could be found in the markets with a little bicycle cart holding their tools or in thimble-sized barbershops. For a few coins, men could get a clean shave with a straight-edge razor. I think my curiosity for these barbers was because my dad owned a little barbershop for over forty years in Phoenix. And like my dad's shop, these tiny Moroccan barbershops always featured men sitting around watching an old TV, probably talking about the news and their kids.

One of the key requirements for achieving a good shave is to first loosen the hair with warm water before you take a razor to your skin. My dad would apply a hot face towel to his customers' faces before shaving them, but if you are shaving other parts of your body, a warm shower will do. And although most of the barbers in the Moroccan shops seemed to use dabs of store-bought paste, I heard rumors that some made their own fancy pastes using various traditional clays of the region. This shaving gel, made with Moroccan kitchen staples such as orange blossom honey and olive oil, incorporates rhassoul clay into the mix, creating a silky potion that's perfect for silky skin. If you want to get extra luxurious, add the optional neroli or rose essential oil for added fragrance. I haven't bought shaving gel for myself since using this recipe.

Makes about ½ cup

¼ cup olive oil

2 tablespoons unscented liquid castile soap

2 tablespoons runny orange blossom honey

1 teaspoon vegetable glycerin

1 teaspoon rhassoul clay

10 drops neroli or rose essential oil (optional)

Small plastic squeeze bottle with lid (a recycled honey bear bottle is perfect)

Put all the ingredients in a small nonmetal bowl and mix them together using a small wooden spoon. Using a funnel, transfer the mixture to the soft squeeze bottle. Use just the same as you would any shaving cream.

TEPEZCOHUITE
HONEY MASK

My first experience with tepezcohuite (*Mimosa tenuiflora*) was in Guatemala many years ago. There was a little botanica in the city of Antigua that was well-stocked with herbal remedies, handmade soaps, and natural beauty products, all made with local ingredients. Traditionally known for its regenerative properties, the bark from this little shrub is used in many products specifically for the skin. I bought some soap and bark pieces.

The soap made a great face wash, but it was the bark that I loved most! I ground the bark to a fine powder using my molcajete and simply mixed it with water to use as a face mask. After using the mask twice a week for a month, I noticed that the sunspots on my face were beginning to fade. This miraculous plant has the ability to promote youthful skin and heal a wide range of skin problems, especially burns. Mixed with honey instead of water, this mask is still one of my absolute favorites!

Makes 1 mask

1 tablespoon tepezcohuite powder
1 tablespoon runny honey

In a small bowl, mix the ingredients with a small spoon. It will seem like it's not coming together at first, but be patient and continue stirring. Once it looks like brownie batter, it's done!

To use, apply the mask with your fingertips to a clean, dry face, being mindful not to get it too close to your eyes. Allow the mask to sit on your skin for at least 15 minutes. Rinse and towel dry your face. You can use this mask up to 3 times a week.

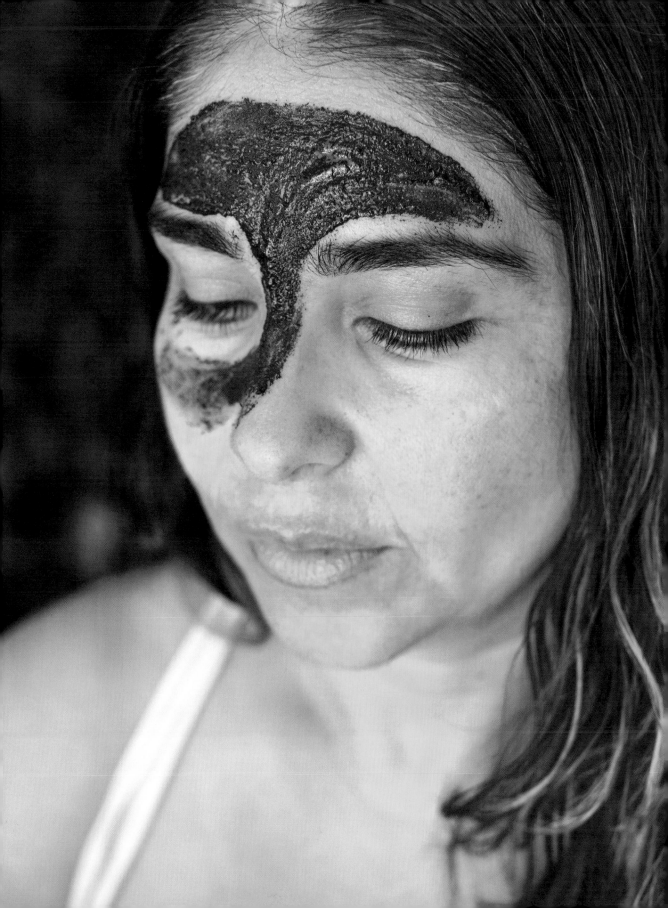

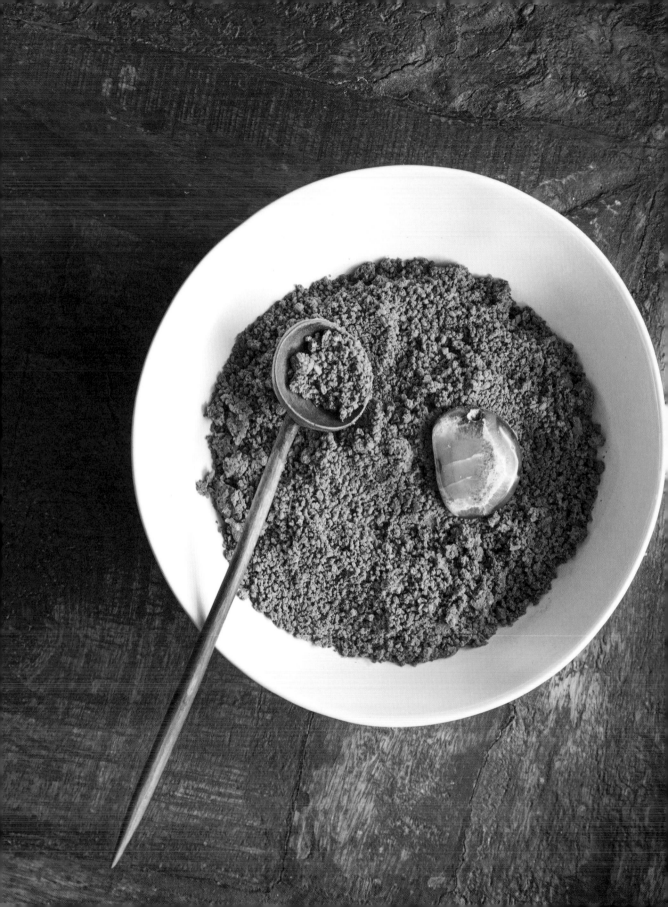

SEDONA BATH SOAK

When I was a child, our family would drive to Sedona during Phoenix summers to escape the heat and spend the day at Oak Creek Canyon. I loved playing in the creek with my siblings, going fishing with my dad, and having lunch by the water. Now that I am an adult, I can see why Sedona is considered the New Age capital of the world. It is a spiritually captivating place that Native peoples inhabited and cherished long before it was said to be connected to the Earth's chakra system.

This bath soak recipe is designed to help relieve sore muscles and is delicately scented with juniper berry essential oil to mimic the twisted juniper trees found throughout the area. The carnelian gemstone added at the end infuses your bath soak, helping circulate vital energy to your center, just like Sedona itself.

Makes 2½ cups (for about 5 baths)

¼ cup red clay
1 cup Epson salt
1 cup baking soda
¼ cup sweet almond oil
10 drops juniper berry essential oil
1 small carnelian gemstone
20-ounce glass jar

Put all the ingredients except for the carnelian gemstone in the bowl and mix with a wooden spoon. Add the carnelian gemstone to the mixture to infuse into the salt. Store the mixture in a glass jar with a lid and label.

To use your bath soak, draw a warm bath, placing a handful of the mixture into the water to dissolve, leaving the gemstone in the jar. Soak for 20 minutes. Keep in mind that pigmented clays can stain white towels, robes, and rugs, so plan accordingly. Gently pat your skin dry.

ROOTED FOOT SCRUB

On a visit to a Guatemalan coffee plantation, my daughter found small treasures such as bright flowers, coffee berries, and special rocks. When our trip ended and it was time to fly back home, we got to the airport, where a customs agent asked if we had any plants, seeds, archeological items, cigars, or other prohibited items in our luggage. I quickly replied no when my daughter, who was five or six at the time, interrupted saying she had "lots of rocks" in her suitcase. Now, border crossings always give me slight anxiety, so this rock declaration gave me instant heart pains. Unbeknownst to me, my daughter had stashed several pumice stones in her bag and in her pockets! And because they were so lightweight, I didn't notice it. We left them with the customs agent, and to this day, whenever I use pumice stone I think of that moment.

Pumice is the result of volcanic eruptions, which is why my daughter had collected so many of the stones. We were staying in Antigua, which has three volcanoes in its vicinity. Volcanoes, as they relate to our own being, represent upward challenges and the goals we wish to aspire to. And although their lava is connected to the element of Fire, volcanoes also harness the power of Earth by reminding us to go deep within, just like the inner workings of the volcano.

Finely ground pumice makes an eco-friendly foot scrub that when applied as ritual, allows us to slow down and acknowledge the feet that keep us steady and rooted.

1 cup fine ground pumice

¼ cup fractionated coconut oil

1 tablespoon castile soap

5 drops tangerine essential oil

4 drops grapefruit essential oil

2 drops geranium essential oil

3 drops cypress essential oil

10-ounce glass jar

Place all the ingredients in a small bowl. Stir with a spoon until everything is well combined. Transfer to the jar and label.

To use the foot scrub, I like to do these steps in my bathtub for easy cleanup. Fill a small basin with warm water and place it in your shower or bathtub. Soak your feet for about 5 minutes in the basin. Empty the water. Then, sitting on the edge of your bathtub or shower bench, massage 1 tablespoon of the scrub into each foot, focusing on the areas where dry skin is most prominent. Rinse and dry your feet.

SPIRITUAL WORK WITH EARTH

MOTHER EARTH ROSE MALA

Red roses are symbolic of love felt at the deepest levels. Their fragrance assists us in feeling calm and grounded while awakening our capacity for self-love. Malas are prayer tools made with 108 beads, which is considered a holy number in Indian spirituality. Additionally, many cultures and religions use prayer beads including Christianity, Islam, and Buddhism. The practice of praying with beads increases our focus, and reciting a mantra or prayer and simply wearing a mala can remind us of our goals and intentions. However, using beads created with rose petals is a unique feminine tribute to the Divine Mother, Mother Earth herself.

Although red is associated with our root chakra, you can use any color rose petal to create this mala. You simply need time and patience.

Makes 1 mala

2 ounces dried red rose petals

Water (preferably spring water)

Rose essential oil (optional)

Complementary store-bought beads (optional)

Thick sewing needles

Beading string

Jewelry fasteners (optional)

Put the dried rose petals in a cast-iron or enamel pot on the stovetop. Add enough water to cover the petals, bring the mixture to a boil, and then turn down the heat to a gentle simmer. Cook uncovered for several hours, stirring occasionally until the petals are broken down, adding more water if needed. When the petals start to turn dark brown, they are done.

(continued)

Put the mixture into a blender and pulse until you have a paste. Next, line a strainer with cheesecloth and strain the petals, squeezing out as much water as possible with your hands. Put the cooked rose petals in a small bowl and add a few drops of the rose oil, if using, and knead the petals like dough. Once the mixture is the consistency of clay, form small balls about the size of a marble, as the balls will shrink after drying. The result will vary depending on humidity and the type of rose petals you use. Keep note of how many beads your recipe yields should you choose to make a mala with 108 beads.

Taking your needles, pierce the center of each rose bead to create a hole for your string. Depending on the length of your needles, you should be able to fit 3 to 5 beads on each needle. Place the pierced beads on a plate or tray and put them somewhere warm to dry. Once they are completely dry, remove the beads from the needles. String your beads onto the beading string, adding complementary beads if desired. Finish the mala with jewelry fasteners, or just tie the ends with a simple knot.

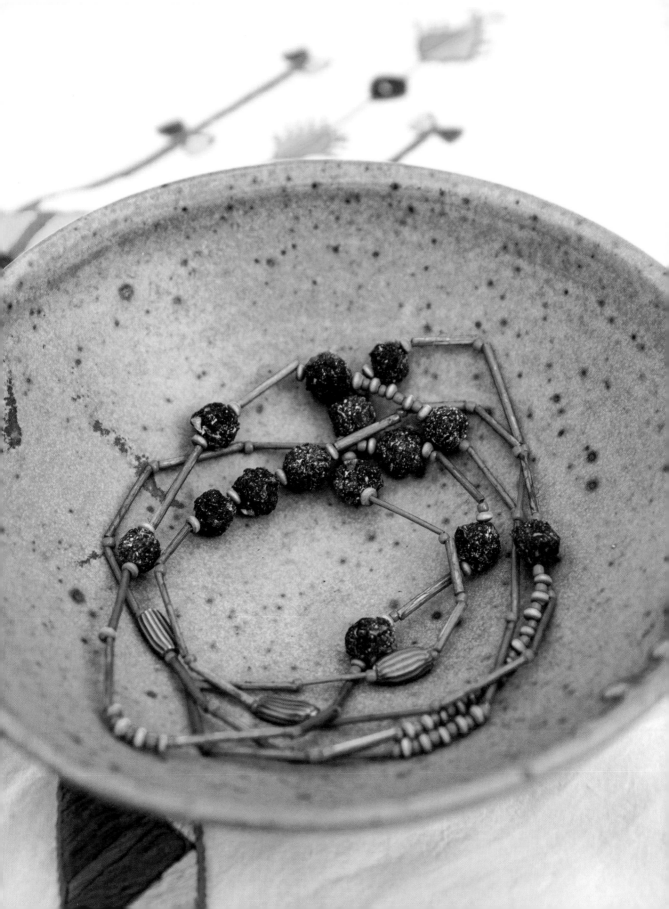

COOKING WITH EARTHENWARE

One of humankind's most important innovations is cookware made from Earth. Some of the best meals I've ever prepared were cooked in clay vessels picked up at estate sales, thrift stores, or my travels abroad. Each one offers a different attribute to the end dish depending on the vessel, lending subtle earthy flavors to stews while keeping the dish warm well after it leaves the flame. I have earthenware I only use for rice, others for beans, some for Moroccan dishes, and one clay comal that I only use for roasting chiles. Once you go down the earthenware rabbit hole, it becomes a slight obsession.

Cooking in or with clay vessels is such a simple way to connect with Earth as you are quite literally cooking with Earth! With so many clay vessels handcrafted around the world, it's a special way to bring your ancestral traditions into your daily life with food. Just be sure to research the type of vessel you will be using as there are a few factors that will help you with a successful dish, such as curing it or preventing cracking due to sudden temperature changes.

One of my favorite earthenware pieces is the humble *olla*, which is a Mexican clay pot used mostly for cooking beans. I once had a friend ask why I would make beans from scratch in my olla when I could easily buy them canned and save time. The truth is, beans are comfort food for me, and eating them prepared this traditional way is usually saved for lazy Sundays when the olla has time to permeate the house with a smell of delicious broth and ancestral taste memories.

FRIJOLES DE LA OLLA

Here is my recipe for pinto beans cooked in a Mexican clay pot with a few other basic ingredients. Epazote is a Mexican herb used often when cooking beans to help make them more digestible and to infuse the broth with a unique flavor profile. In my opinion, dried epazote does not offer the same results, so if you cannot find fresh epazote, just omit it.

About 6 cups

1 pound pinto beans, picked through and rinsed
1 white onion, peeled, left whole, and scored with a knife
1 head of garlic
1 tablespoon olive oil
4 fresh epazote leaves
Sea salt
Medium-sized Mexican clay olla

Place the beans in the olla and cover them with 3 inches of water. Allow the beans to soak overnight or for at least a few hours. Drain off the soaking water (I like to water my plants with this). Return the soaked beans to the olla and add the onion, garlic, olive oil, epazote, and enough water to cover the beans by 3 to 4 inches.

Place the olla on a fire source, such as a gas stove, butane tabletop burner, or outdoor firepit. Bring the water to boil and then reduce to simmer. Cook the beans for 1 to 2 hours, adding more water if necessary. The time will vary depending on the age of the beans, how long they soaked, and the strength of the fire. They should be firm yet tender when they are almost done. Add sea salt to taste and simmer for 20 to 30 more minutes more to season the beans. Remove the onion, garlic, and epazote with a slotted spoon and add salt if needed. I was always taught to give the beans a little mash with a potato masher to create a richer broth before serving. They taste best with warm corn tortillas.

EARTHLY DELIGHTS ANOINTING OIL

How do you define abundance? When I was reworking my abundance mindset, one obstacle that kept blocking my progress was my belief that spiritual people could not have nice things. Somewhere in my upbringing and strengthened by my cultural experiences, I learned that being a spiritual person meant I should not have a nice car, live in a nice area, or have money in my account. I was far into adulthood when I decided that I could no longer allow other people to define what abundance looked like to me.

I realized I didn't feel guilty for having abundant health, spiritual wealth, or rich friendships, but the guilt I had for desiring money went deep. I decided to redefine the word *abundance* for myself. My new definition included core virtues like stability, freedom, and the opportunity to give to others without neglecting my own needs. And then I gave myself permission to desire whatever I wanted, even if they were earthly delights. So many opportunities opened for me after that clarification. And so, to continue that momentum, I enjoy dabbing this blend on my wrists when I am doing abundance work. While smelling it on my skin, I say thank you to Creator for all the abundance I have and for what is coming my way.

This blend is made with Peru balsam from El Salvador, which when blended with fresh ginger and dark patchouli, harnesses the earth's abundant energy, creating an anointing oil that welcomes in prosperity. I often wear this simply as my perfume.

Makes one perfume bottle

15 drops Peru balsam essential oil

10 drops patchouli essential oil

10 drops ginger essential oil

2 tablespoons jojoba oil

1–2 ounce glass perfume bottle or dark glass bottle

Put all the ingredients in the bottle, add the lid, and gently mix by rolling the bottle between the palms of your hand, infusing it with good intentions.

To use ritually, apply a small amount of the anointing oil to your wrists, heart, or third eye as part of your daily gratitude or abundance practice.

WATERING THE EARTH WITH MOONTIME BLOOD

I never thought I would miss my monthly moontime, but now as I enter menopause, soon I will not be able to water the earth as I have for years with my moontime blood. In 2012, I embraced using a menstrual cup to capture my flow, which was relatively heavy. As I result, I really got to know my body differently through my menstrual blood. The color, the amount, how it changed when I did my steams. Seeing this blood through new eyes gave me an appreciation for my cycle and my blood in a way I had not embraced in the past. Among many ancient cultures around the world, it is believed that menstrual blood carries very powerful energy. In my own experience, I was taught that I could not participate in sweat lodge ceremony because women are in their full power during our moontime. Suddenly, I felt strange, discarding this magical substance, and started researching rituals in which our blood was returned to Earth.

I learned that offerings of moontime blood are cross-cultural. Ancient practices of offering blood to Earth for blessings or simply to celebrate womanhood are found all over the world. But so many of these practices were deemed primitive or shameful, and they disappeared with the rise of pads, tampons, and patriarchy. The first time I "watered" earth with my blood, I felt very connected to the tree I had placed it under. Since then, doing so has helped me reclaim my power during this time while nourishing the ground that supports me.

It is easiest to water earth using blood caught in a menstrual cup, cloth pad, or period panties such as Thinx. Listen to your spirit to see which method works best for you. Also, no need to go outside if you do not feel comfortable doing so or do not have access to Nature. A houseplant will do just fine. Our moontime blood is full of nutrients that plants love, so they will benefit from your offering as much as an oak tree in your backyard.

If you use cloth pads, you already rinse or allow them to soak in water prior to laundering them. That crimson liquid is the water that you want to use as your offering. If you use menstrual cups, you can simply pour it into a little jar and offer it to your houseplants or pour it directly into the ground. Sometimes, I choose to water all my plants with this magic, so I dilute it in my watering can to nourish all the plants in my home.

There's no right or wrong way in offering your moontime blood back to the Earth. I usually close my eyes for a moment and simply set an intention or offer gratitude for keeping me grounded.

AMETHYST HIGH VIBRATIONAL PERFUME: GROUNDING WITH GEMSTONES

To me, grounding is touching Mother Earth's soil, rocks, and waters with our feet to stay connected to her vital force. Much like an electrical appliance, when you are truly grounded, your energy is balanced. When I was a practicing massage therapist, I could always sense who was physically "grounded" simply by touching their feet. The ones who squirmed and giggled at the slightest touch were the ones who rarely touched the Earth. But the ones who had thick skin and worn-looking feet were rarely ticklish. These were the ones who spent more time grounding barefoot outside in their yards or on adventures.

Coming in contact with Earth on a regular basis nurtures our physical being much like the bonding that happens in skin-to-skin contact with newborn babies. We need to bond with the Earth to feel her energy and foster a healthy relationship. If you are unable to get outside on a regular basis, you can still connect with the Earth by incorporating more gemstones and minerals into your daily lives.

For instance, black tourmaline is one of the most grounding crystals. It can transduce energy, making it one of the most efficient minerals for absorbing electromagnetic radiation. Meaning, it's a great crystal to have near your computer and other electronics. Rose quartz (one of my favorites), on the other hand, is a wonderful crystal to scatter around your space to attract feelings of calm.

For next-level grounding, I uplift and rebalance my energy with roll-on perfumes created with crystal chips and essentials oils. They are simple to make, carry high vibrations, and allow me to start my day with the intention of connecting to Earth before I even leave the house. Here is an elixir for balance, protection, and third eye power.

Makes one rollerball

10 to 20 amethyst chips
6 drops lavender essential oil
4 drops bergamot essential oil
4 drops frankincense essential oil
3 drops marjoram essential oil
2 drops lemon essential oil
2 drops sweet orange essential oil
Fractionated coconut oil
1- to 2-ounce glass bottle with rollerball

Take the roller off your bottle. Place your amethyst chips inside. Add all the essential oils. Top off the bottle with the fractionated coconut oil. Place the roller back on the bottle and shake gently to mix. Label.

To use your perfume, apply it to your wrist points, temples, and collarbone.

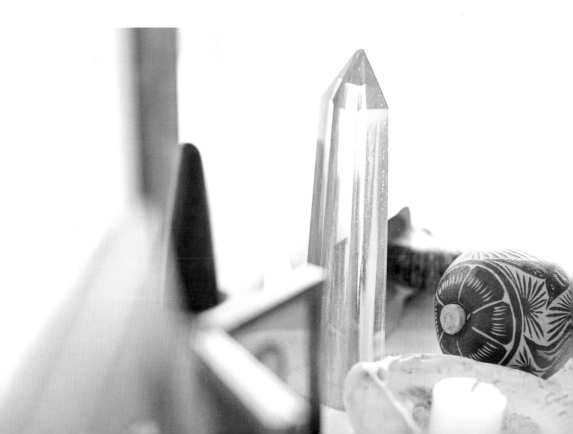

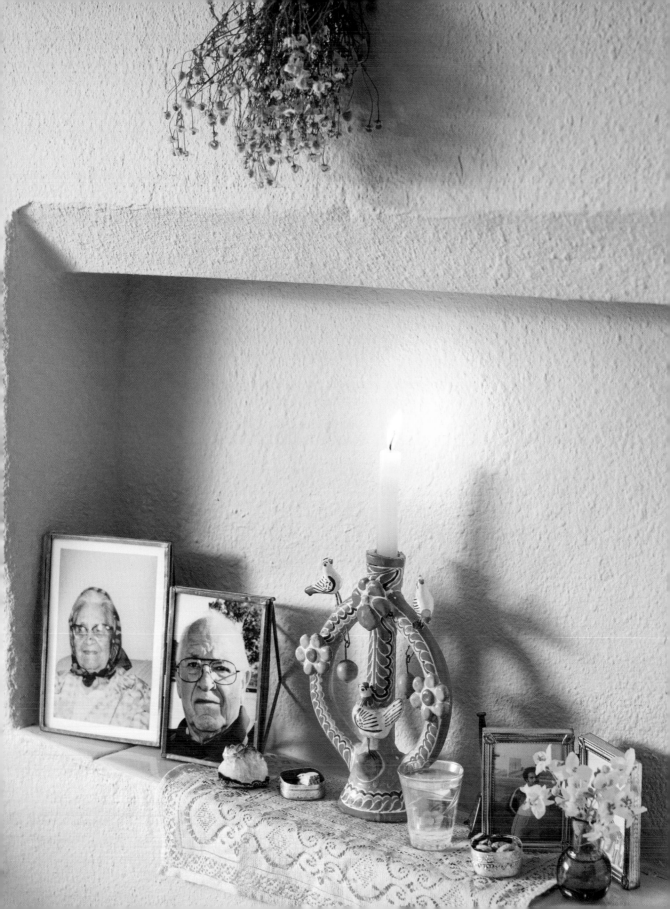

CREATING AN ANCESTOR ALTAR

The Earth element is one of downward moving energy, going so deep that it reaches far into our ancestral roots. As an ancestral worker, one of the most important tools I suggest to my clients is the healing use of an ancestor altar. Creating an ancestor altar is a beautiful way to honor those who came before you and to invoke them for guidance and support in your daily activities.

Cultures all over the world create ancestor shrines or altars to show reverence to those who have passed on. In my own home, I've always kept an ancestor altar up year-round. My ancestor altar is a dedicated space where I can go to communicate and receive messages from those who played important roles in my life or to connect with the ones I never got to know.

Every culture, religion, and tradition is unique in how it shows reverence to ancestors. So, I give the upcoming assembly suggestions merely as a starting point. I encourage you to do your homework by digging deeper into your lineage to see how you can personalize your altar to best represent your own bloodline. I also believe that there is no right or wrong way to assemble an ancestor altar, as I feel our ancestors are grateful that we are taking the time to honor them in such a sacred manner. Lastly, for many, we have had influential people in our lives who are not related to us by blood. I love honoring these people as well on my ancestor altar because I believe they are my ancestors in spirit.

(continued)

Altar Space: The location for your altar is dependent on space and privacy. Some people have a large cabinet or side table to set up their altar, while others are limited by space or do not feel comfortable having their altar in plain view of company. Do what feels best for you and your situation, keeping in mind that it's the intention that is the most important element. I've suggested to those with limited space or privacy concerns to create altars in cigar boxes or shoeboxes so they can take them out to pray and store them when needed.

Altar Cloth: I was taught to and prefer to use a white piece of cloth as an altarpiece to anchor my altar space because white helps invite the spirits in. However, any natural cloth that resonates with you will do.

Candle: I use white candles to ignite when speaking with my ancestors. Be sure to place your candles where they will be safe, and never leave them burning when you are not home.

Libations: As an offering, I always have a little glass of fresh water for my ancestors, and sometimes when invoking a specific ancestor that loved a certain libation, I may leave a tiny glass of rum or tequila for them.

Photos: If you have the privilege of having photos of your ancestors, this is the perfect space to honor them. I was taught, however, that you should never have a picture that includes you or any other living people in any of the photos of the ancestors you wish to honor.

Offerings: This is where you can get very creative, and as mentioned before, add offerings to your altar that resonate with your bloodline. Sometimes I place a cigar, blue corn seeds, medicinal roots, and even okra seeds for my husband's African ancestors. Often, I put a baby jar of fresh herbs out if it is something I am cooking with that day as I have one ancestor who loved cooking with fresh herbs.

Aromatics: This is one of my favorite pieces of my altar because I love how the smoke carries my intentions to my ancestors. If you cannot burn incense on your altar space, you can create my recipe for Agua de Florida (see page 51) to spritz on your altar or to refresh your altar when needed.

Call on Their Names: I was taught that after a loved one passes, you should not ask them for help for at least one year after their transition so that they may get accustomed to the spirit realm. When invoking my own ancestors each morning, I ring a small bell and state the following to protect my energy and space.

Good morning, Ancestors! I call on you (state their names) and all my ancestors who are spiritually well and resonating at the highest frequency to guide me and support me today.

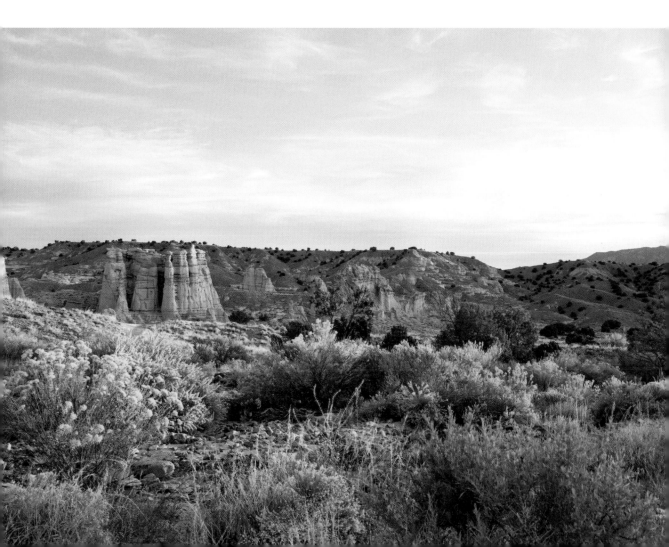

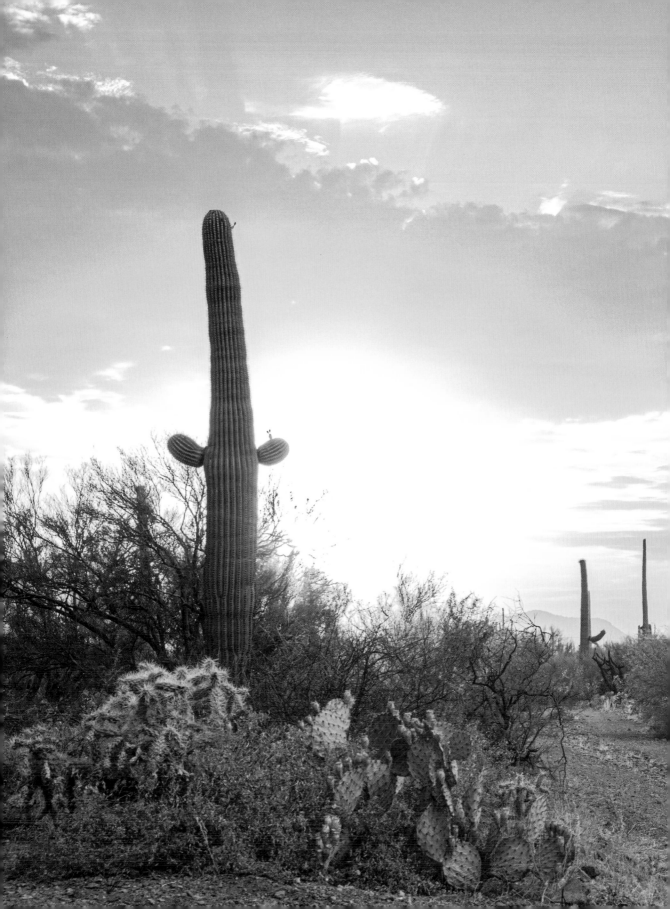

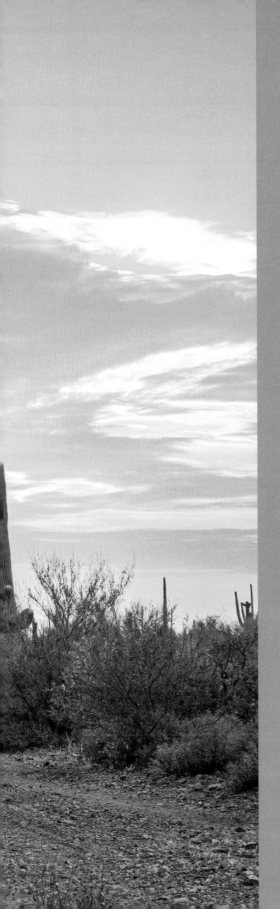

159 ◇ FIRE

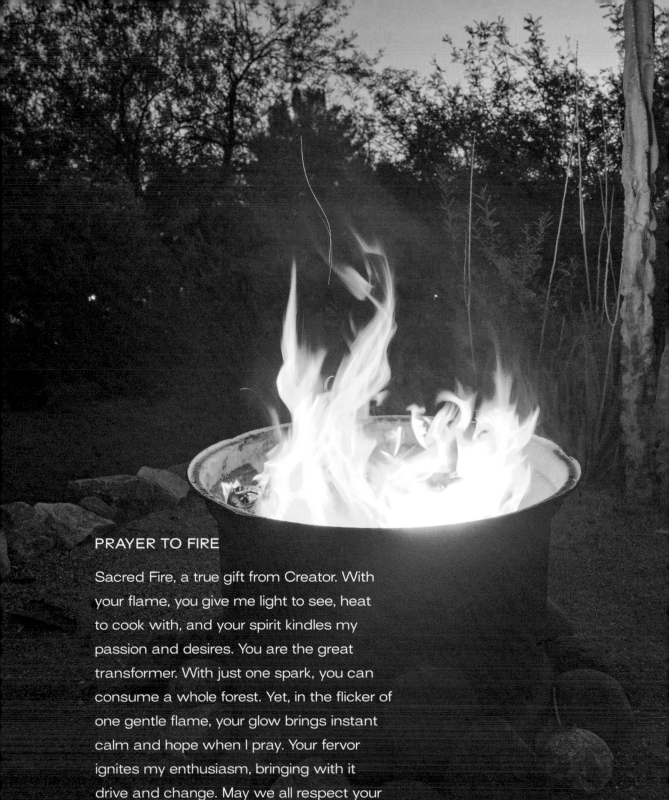

PRAYER TO FIRE

Sacred Fire, a true gift from Creator. With
your flame, you give me light to see, heat
to cook with, and your spirit kindles my
passion and desires. You are the great
transformer. With just one spark, you can
consume a whole forest. Yet, in the flicker of
one gentle flame, your glow brings instant
calm and hope when I pray. Your fervor
ignites my enthusiasm, bringing with it
drive and change. May we all respect your
energy and use it for awareness.

FIRE FOR INNER HARMONY

THE BEAUTY OF FIRE

SPIRITUAL WORK WITH FIRE

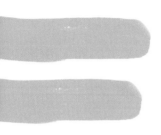

AN ALCHEMIST BY DESIGN, FIRE IS TRANSMUTATIVE.

Fire. Whether you are relaxing around a campfire, hypnotized by its flames or listening closely to the news of a nearby brushfire, Fire captures everyone's attention. An alchemist by design, Fire is transmutative. The energy behind its flame is one of mystery, change, and destruction. Nonetheless, after even the greatest of destruction comes renewal and rebirth as demonstrated by the mythological phoenix. Illuminating people with its medicine, Fire is the strongest and most powerful of all the elements, and it is something that I was taught to respect.

Throughout my life, I have witnessed Fire keepers tending to Fire for ceremony or dance. Fire keepers are designated community members upholding the age-old tradition of keeping a fire strong and hot, working with it, praying to it, and showing it utmost respect. Keeping the fire strong is not simply for heating stones that may be used in a sweat lodge or providing light and warmth for a dance. It is also representative of the spiritual energy of the ceremony or gathering, which is why a fire needs to remain strong and must never die out until the end of the ceremony. Depending on the tribe or tradition, sacred aromatics may be placed on the hot rocks heated by this sacred flame. This exchange is an offering and a prayer of gratitude. It is a reminder that when you work with Fire to see it as a living entity.

Nourishing my body with the bright Fire of the sun is not only one of my beauty secrets for glowing skin, but it is also a key to good gut health. Eating daily an array of colorful fruits and vegetables is nutritionally healing, and their colors transport me to memories of sunny days. It's no wonder that when many of us experience high levels of stress or consume too many processed foods, we can send our digestive systems into high alert. Nutrient-rich plant foods infused with the sun not only invigorate our metabolism, but they can also energize our spirit.

When you eat a diet of diverse plants, you are in essence eating the sun's energy—Fire energy. And harnessing the actual element to cook with helps you connect with Fire in an ancestral way also sparking your inner Fire.

If you listen to how people describe others who appear healthy, they often reference the sun and the qualities of Fire. "She has sparkles in her eyes, beautiful glowing skin, and her hair is wild and sun-kissed." There are many notable benefits of receiving sunlight exposure each day including its ability to boost our body's vitamin D supply and elevating our mood. To get that inner and outer glow, consider taking a sun break each day to soak up some sunlight, promoting an overall sense of well-being and generating beauty from within. Nonetheless, every person and their geographical location is different, so use moderation and common sense. And if you receive too much sun, be sure to try the Sol Soother!

Fire reminds us to approach life and one another with keen awareness and great respect. It teaches us how to move through difficult life transitions with its flames of insight and guidance. A provoker of change, Grandfather Fire is a wise and sacred energy that awakens our hearts and helps us move through times of great transformation. It is a powerful energy connecting us to enlightenment. A source of power and strength, Fire gives us the courage we may need while its warmth fuels our desires and passions. When we are feeling lethargic, lazy, or creatively depleted, bringing more Fire into our life raises the vibration of our energy.

And while Air and Water are both clearing and cleansing elements, Fire is transforming. Working spiritually with the energy of Fire is beneficial when you seek purposeful action, change, or renewal. It encourages us like the sun, that we too can radiate light, warmth, and creative energy for ourselves and to those around us.

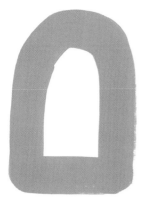

FIRE
FOR INNER
HARMONY

ELECTUARY FOR DIGESTIVE FIRE

Warming herbs such as ginger have widely been used for the digestive system, helping with ailments such as an upset stomach, nausea, and indigestion. While studying Ayurvedic cooking, I learned that several of my common kitchen spices could be eaten to increase the digestion of food and raise the metabolic process in our bodies. This is valuable because a strong metabolism causes more heat in the body, which helps with the digestion process and is believed to help break down and transform food. This action is called *agni*, the fire of digestion. Hence, consuming the correct herbs and spices can "feed" agni and strengthen its energy, thus allowing for healthy ingestion of nutrients. The general signs that you may have a weak digestive fire are experiencing a poor appetite, feeling sleepy after meals, having excessive gas, and feeling heavy or lethargic.

An electuary is simply a mixture of powdered herbs and spices combined with honey to make a thick paste that you can take by the spoonful or add to warm water. I have made electuaries using fresh plant material such as the zest of a lemon or grated ginger, but for the most part, they are traditionally made using dried powdered herbs and spices for a longer shelf life. Any of these spices are great for digestion and can be used on their own or blended to make your own special combination. It's a straightforward method and a tasty way to introduce more Fire into your body.

(continued)

Amount varies

Anise seeds

Black pepper

Cardamom pods

Cayenne

Cinnamon

Coriander seeds

Cumin seeds

Dill seeds

Fennel seeds

Ginger

Runny honey

This recipe makes one small jar and is very flexible. You will need about 4 teaspoons of ground spices and approximately ½ cup of honey.

To begin, first decide which spices you would like to use from the above list, choosing one single spice or several spices for your creation. Don't worry about exact measurements, but aim for roughly 4 teaspoons total. If any of your chosen spices are whole, you will first need to grind them using a mortar and pestle. Once you have your blend of ground spices, place them in your jar and begin adding honey to create a thick paste, mixing and adjusting the honey if you want a thinner or sweeter electuary. Label the jar.

To use the electuary, take one small teaspoonful before meals to enkindle your agni.

TRUE SUN-DRIED TOMATOES

When I was a little girl, our family had several green grapevines growing along a fence in our backyard. Each year for many years, my dad would harvest the grapes to make green grape jelly and sun-dried raisins. He would use two wooden sawhorses with an old screen door on top and place the grapes on the screen, covering them with netting to protect from birds. Days later, we had pounds of raisins. This is a perfect example of how easy it is to preserve food by harnessing the sun's energy.

There are many methods to make sun-dried tomatoes, but something about drying tomatoes using the actual sun not only feels more authentic but it's also slow food, which reminds us to be patient and honor the process. Drying tomatoes at home is relatively easy, but there are a few factors to keep in mind such as temperature, good air circulation, and humidity. The ideal temperature for sun-drying tomatoes is 85 degrees, with higher temperatures being even better. If you live in a high-humidity environment, it may be more difficult as the humidity will prevent moisture from leaving the tomatoes.

Amount varies

Several pounds of Roma or cherry tomatoes, uniform in size
Sea salt

Slice the tomatoes in half lengthwise and lay them cut side up in a single layer on a drying tray, such as a large cooling rack. Season them well with sea salt. Cover the tray with cheesecloth and place it in a sunny spot with good air circulation. Leave the tomatoes outside for several days until their texture is no longer tacky and resembles plump raisins. Store the dried tomatoes in vacuum-sealed bags, freezer bags, or jars in the refrigerator or freezer. Or, you can seal them in a sterile canning jar, packed with olive oil.

ISIS SUN TEA

Isis is an Egyptian goddess associated with the sun and is believed to be a true messenger of solar power. Often depicted with a solar disk on her head, she is known as the Radiant Goddess or Lady of the House of Fire and is a protective goddess who uses magic spells to help others in need. Responsible for the rising of the sun, she is said to love flowers, water, and honey, which are three of the ingredients needed to make this delicious hibiscus solar tea.

Here in the Southwest, many of us of Mexican descent grew up drinking a tart hibiscus beverage known as *agua de flor de jamaica*, made from the dried calyces of the roselle flower. It was and still is one of my favorite beverages to enjoy on a really hot day, and it doesn't hurt that it is full of antioxidants. The main ingredient in Isis Sun Tea is the calyces from the *Hibiscus sabdariffa* shrub, also known as roselle or by its common name, hibiscus. The calyces can be found at most international grocers. When I want to channel more Fire, more sun, and more magical Isis energy, I remember to place my sun tea jar of hibiscus out to infuse on a bright sunny day.

Makes about 12 cups

½ cup dried hibiscus flowers
2 tablespoons dried rose petals
Few sprigs of fresh mint
12 cups water
Honey

Put the hibiscus flowers, rose petals, and mint in a square of cheesecloth or a nut milk bag, making a little bundle. Add the herb bundle to a glass gallon jar. Fill with the water. Place the jar out in the direct sun for a few hours. Remove the herb bundle and sweeten the tea with honey to taste.

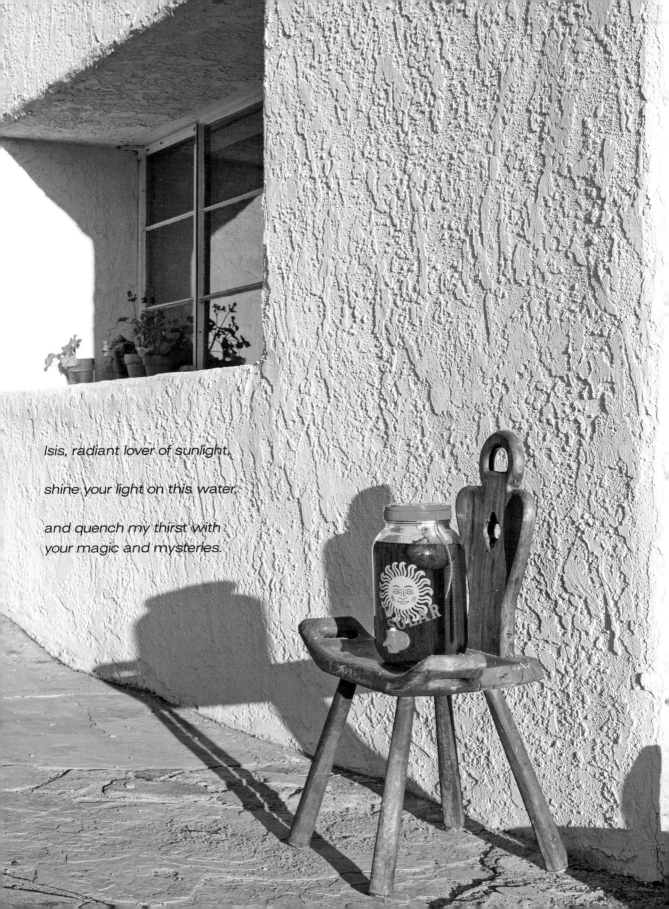

Isis, radiant lover of sunlight,

shine your light on this water,

and quench my thirst with
your magic and mysteries.

BORAGE TWO WAYS

Sometimes we overheat from the effects of too much Fire. This can be felt physically when experiencing a fever or emotionally when under stressful conditions. I myself have felt my "blood rise" during periods of emotional distress, which then puts physical stress on my adrenal glands. One of my favorite herbs to take during these times is borage (*Borago officinalis*), for its useful properties in helping restore and refresh adrenal glands, thus helping cool our inner Fire.

I especially love using fresh borage because it is easy to grow from seed, it yields a lot of plant material, and the fresh leaves are reminiscent of cucumber—one of my favorite flavors. The leaves and purple flowers can be used straight from the garden in beverages and salads, and I truly believe it is an important culinary herb to include in your home healing garden.

When fresh leaves are prepared as a cooling restorative tonic, they infuse the water with a delicate refreshing flavor. But, when made as a hot infusion, the flavor along with the medicinal properties intensifies. Borage leaves make wonderful adaptogenic tonics, which is a gentle reminder that this is herbal medicine not to be taken daily, but only after times of stress to help restore the health of your adrenal glands.

BORAGE RESTORATIVE WATER
Makes about 8 cups

One handful fresh borage leaves and flowers
Lemon, thinly sliced into circles or half-moons
8 cups water

Lightly bruise the borage leaves with the back of a wooden spoon. Place the borage leaves, lemon slices, and water into a large pitcher or jar. Allow them to infuse for 15 to 20 minutes. Serve at room temperature or chilled.

BORAGE HOT NERVINE INFUSION

Makes about 4 cups

One cup fresh borage leaves and flowers
4 cups water
Honey

Using the back of a wooden spoon, gently bruise the borage leaves. Put the leaves and flowers in a tea infuser or French press. Boil the water and allow it to cool slightly. Pour the hot water over the borage and cover it, allowing the herbs to infuse for 3 minutes. Strain and enjoy your infusion, adding honey to taste.

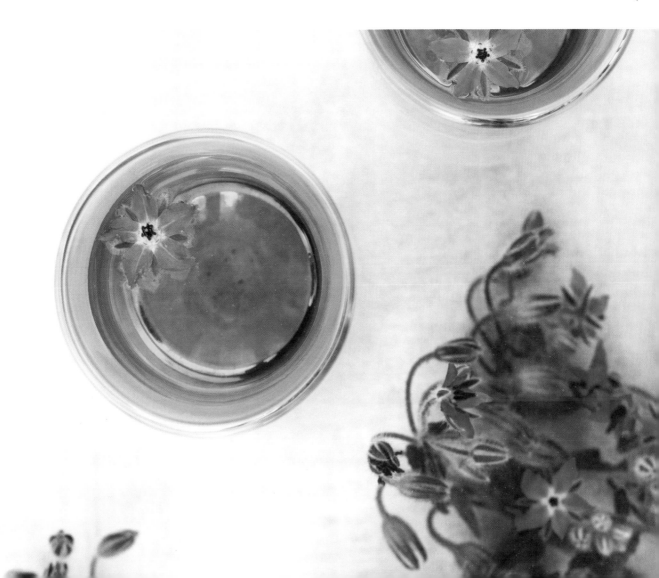

GINGER FIRE
HONEY CHEWS

Ginger is one of my all-time favorite anti-inflammatory foods. Packed with a lot of Fire energy, it has the ability to reduce inflammation in the body, helping to relieve pain such as menstrual cramps, arthritis, and headache. I find it so interesting how hot, warm, spicy foods such as ginger can work as an anti-inflammatory given the breakdown of the word *inflammatory*—to be inflamed, in flames.

I enjoy eating candied ginger as a treat but hate all the sugar. Making them with honey eases my mind, as honey does contain trace vitamins and minerals, and it soothes my throat as well. Normally, when I teach how to prepare herbal remedies using honey, I advise to never heat raw honey over 100°F so to not change the enzymatic composition of the honey. However, for this recipe, the honey is used solely as a natural sweetener, so I suggest runny honey versus raw solid honey. These chews are easy to make, though they do take a lot of time to simmer and dry. I like to prepare them on a day off when I can start first thing in the morning.

Makes about 25 chews

1 pound fresh organic ginger, scrubbed well
1½ cup runny honey
1½ cup water

Slice the ginger into thin slices, about ⅛ of an inch. Place the ginger slices in your saucepan and add the honey and water. Bring the mixture to a simmer, reduce heat, cover with a lid, and simmer for 30 minutes. Remove the lid and continue simmering for 30 more minutes. Check the ginger for tenderness by piercing a piece with a small knife. If it pierces easily, remove the saucepan from heat. The honey syrup should be reduced by half at this point. Strain the ginger pieces by using a fine mesh strainer, saving the honey syrup for other uses, such as sweetening teas and drizzling over oatmeal.

Preheat your oven to 200°F. Place the ginger slices on a sheet pan lined with parchment paper and bake 3 to 6 hours (the time depends on the thickness of your ginger slices and how chewy you like your pieces). When ready, remove the ginger slices from the oven, allow them to cool, and store them in the refrigerator.

VEGETARIAN GREEN CHILE SAUCE

The first seventeen summers of my life included spending time in Old Town Albuquerque with my grandmothers in their adobe home, visiting with extended family, and eating lots of food made with green chile. If my parents made the journey to New Mexico late in the summer, that meant we would return home with gunnysacks full of fresh green chiles to roast in our backyard. Roasting green chiles was a family ordeal, with my parents roasting the chiles on the barbecue and me cleaning and bagging roasted chiles by the dozen. It was tedious work, but still one of my favorite memories because of the scent of those chiles. My dad once said that the scent of green chiles being roasted was so powerful that it could even wake up the dead.

Roasting chiles on an open flame adds a flavor profile that tastes ancient and enhances any salsa recipe. If you are able to roast your chiles in an actual wood-fired pit, the smoky flavor will be even more intense, however, a gas or charcoal grill will do. This is one of my favorite ways to connect with Fire—by cooking with it.

(continued)

How to Roast Green Chiles

Start with a hot fire (an outdoor firepit or barbecue) and whole, washed chiles. Place them over the fire, turning them frequently with barbecue tongs, until they are charred and blistered on the outside. After they are roasted, you can let them cool and bag them for later or steam them to peel before storing them, which is what I like to do by following the next steps: Take the chiles from the fire and place them immediately in a paper bag such as a large grocery bag. Close the bag and let them sit for 10 minutes. The heat from the fire and the moisture from the chile will sweat the skin loose.

After 10 minutes, remove the chiles from the bag and scrape the charred skin, peeling it off with a kitchen knife. It will be messy, but the skin should come off easily. Once the charred skin is cleaned off, cut the chile open, and remove the stem and the seeds from the inside. Rinse if needed. Roasted chiles freeze very well.

Makes about 4 cups

2 tablespoons olive oil

½ small onion, minced

3 garlic cloves, minced

2 tablespoons all-purpose flour

2 cups vegetable broth or water

2 cups roasted New Mexico green chile (mild, medium, or hot), chopped

½ teaspoon Mexican oregano

½ teaspoon sea salt

Using a medium saucepan, warm the olive oil over medium heat. Add the onion and garlic, cover, turn the heat down to low, and cook for 3 to 5 minutes until the onion is soft and translucent. Stir in the flour and continue cooking another 1 to 2 minutes. When the flour mixture just begins to color, slowly add the broth or water, stirring constantly to avoid any lumps. Add the green chile, oregano, and salt. Cover the sauce and simmer on low for another 30 minutes. The finished sauce should not be too thick. Dilute it with more broth or water if needed. Taste for seasoning and adjust if necessary. Serve straightaway with Frijoles de la Olla (see page 147), eggs, or warm tortillas.

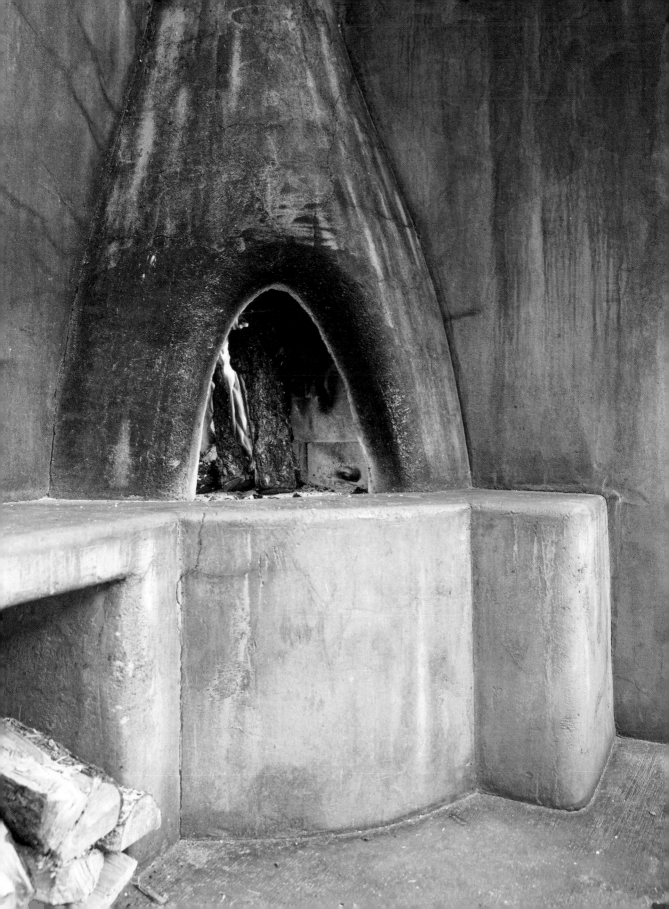

THE
BEAUTY OF
FIRE

HOT FLASH ROLLERBALL

When I first started experiencing hot flashes, I felt like I did when I visited Washington D.C. for the first time in the month of July. I was clammy, hot, needed to get the hair off the back of my neck, and I wanted a cool glass of water. Entering perimenopause was a huge transformation for me, and having hot flashes was one of my first signals. I am still experiencing hot flashes, and they have no rhyme or reason when they show up.

One of the best things I did to tame them was to listen to a friend who had already gone through menopause. She recommended I apply and inhale specific essential oils when I was experiencing a hot flash, and for me, it has been a game changer. There are many blends, with formulations including clary sage and peppermint—both excellent for their hormone-balancing and cooling effects. However, my heart space and emotions also felt hot when I was in the midst of a flash. I would feel anger almost instantly and would have to remind myself that the hot flash was only temporary. That is why I created the blend below, to not only cool my body but to also cool my nervous system as well with rose and jasmine.

Makes one rollerball

12 drops geranium essential oil

8 drops melissa essential oil

4 drops rose essential oil

4 drops jasmine essential oil

Carrier oil (jojoba or fractionated coconut oil work best)

1- to 2-ounce glass bottle with rollerball

(continued)

Add all the essential oils to the glass bottle. Next, using a funnel, add your carrier oil, saving a little space at the top. Add the rollerball and lid and gently roll the bottle between your palms to blend the oils. Label.

To use the rollerball, apply it to your pulse points—inside of your elbows, back of your neck, and your sternum—when needed.

SOL SOOTHER

As much as I love the sun to grow my food, supply me with vitamin D, and keep my city warm year-round, spending too much time under his glow can burn my skin. Everyone is susceptible to sun damage; however, the fairer your skin, the greater your risk for visibly burning your skin after prolonged exposure. That's in part because the melanin present in darker skin tones helps block ultraviolet rays. This does not mean people like me with olive skin aren't at risk for sun damage. It just means that my skin is not as sensitive to the magnificent power of the sun's rays.

If you have ever spent too much time under the Fire of the sun and found yourself with a mild burn, it can feel painful for days afterward. Applying an after-sun spray made with soothing aloe vera and flower botanicals can help reduce inflammation, moisturize your skin, and cool your itchy burn. And because I live in a warm climate where I spend a lot of time outside, I like to have this made and stored in my refrigerator *before* I experience a sunburn so it's ready to go if needed. I also enjoy misting it on my skin even if I am not experiencing a sunburn as it feels really refreshing after a long day outside.

Makes about 1 cup

1 cup water
½ cup dried lavender flowers
¼ cup aloe vera gel (see page 27)
10 drops geranium essential oil
¼ teaspoon vitamin E oil (optional)
8-ounce dark glass bottle with mister

Bring the water to boil in a small saucepan. Turn off the heat and add the lavender flowers. Cover with the lid and infuse 15 to 20 minutes. Using a small mesh strainer, strain the flowers, pressing them with the back of a spoon to release the liquid. Add the aloe vera gel to the bottle. Add the geranium essential oil and vitamin E, if using. Top the bottle off with your lavender water, leaving room for the mister. Cap, shake gently, and label the bottle. Keep the mixture refrigerated until ready to use. To use, mist it on your skin after prolonged sun exposure.

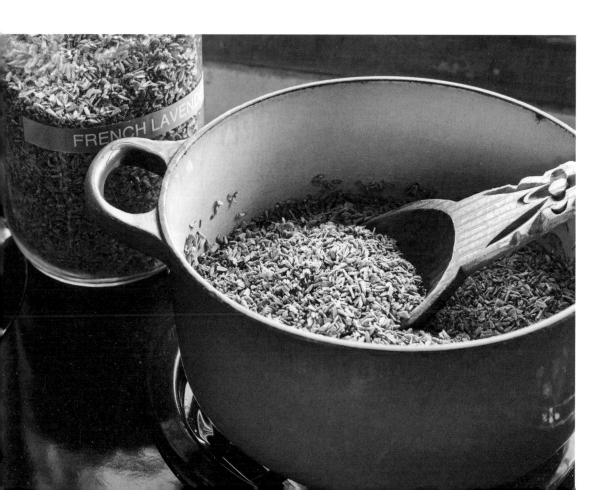

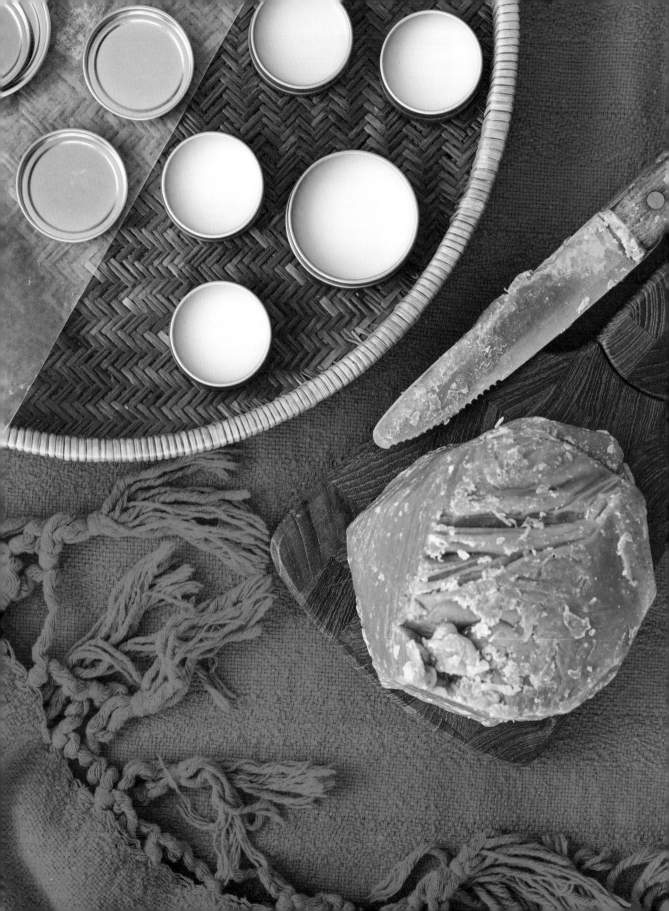

FIERCE TIGRESS
BODY BALM

This hot and spicy topical balm is my version of the tried-and-true Chinese ointment called Tiger Balm, which started showing up in health food stores decades ago for joint pain relief, headaches, and then some. The basic principle behind the ointment is to help move qi and get the blood flowing to areas of pain so healing can take place.

However, although it is recommended as a natural remedy, Tiger Balm does contain petroleum and paraffin. I love its scent and effectiveness, so I created my own version using beeswax, coconut oil, and plenty of essential oils that are beneficial for bringing Fire and warmth to my areas of pain to get my blood flowing. This blend is made with a high dilution of warming essential oils, as it is only meant to be applied to an area of pain. So, even though it smells fierce, please do not slather this on like body butter or get it too close to your eyes.

Makes about 3 ounces

¼ cup solid coconut oil

2 tablespoons beeswax pellets

1 tablespoon menthol crystals

25 drops eucalyptus essential oil

25 drops peppermint essential oil

10 drops cinnamon leaf essential oil

10 drops clove essential oil

10 drops ginger essential oil

10 drops chili seed essential oil

3-ounce glass jar

(continued)

Begin by gently melting the coconut oil, the beeswax pellets, and the menthol crystals in a double boiler (see page 12). While the mixture is melting, measure out your essential oils in a small glass, such as a shot glass. Once the beeswax mixture has melted, turn off the heat and allow it to sit a few minutes to cool slightly. Pour your essential oils into your beeswax mixture and stir it with a wooden chopstick. Immediately pour it into your glass jar. Label.

To use, apply the balm to areas of pain, keeping it away from your eyes. If your mixture thickened too quickly, warm the mixture up briefly to liquify.

STIMULATING RICE BRAN HAIR OIL

I have done a few "big chops" over my life in reflection to what was happening to me personally. After my brother's passing at age twenty, I let go of over a foot of hair in my grief. The same after closing my restaurant during the Great Recession, and again when my father passed while writing this book. Each time was a substantial amount of hair, symbolizing my release of energy and memories.

However, after my second big chop, my hair was the shortest I had ever had it and I couldn't bring myself to grow it back out. That was until Benita's words. Benita was an elder in my community who quietly took me aside one evening and said, "*Mija*, it's time to grow your hair back out. Do everything you can do to make it strong because it represents your path." I gave her the biggest hug and went home that night very emotional. She had given me the spark I needed to grow my hair back long. The next morning, I got to work in the kitchen.

Rice bran and avocado oil are both high in vitamin E, which can promote strong, healthy hair, and rosemary essential oil stimulates the hair follicle to bring more blood flow to the scalp. My hair not only seemed to grow faster when using the mask weekly but it was also really shiny for days after using the blend. I still use this recipe at least once a month to nourish my hair, and when I do, I always think of Benita, who is an ancestor now.

Makes about ½ cup

5 drops rosemary essential oil
¼ cup rice bran oil
¼ cup avocado oil
4-ounce dark glass bottle with dropper

Add the rosemary essential oil to the bottle. Add the rice bran and avocado oils, leaving room for the dropper. Cap with the dropper and roll the bottle gently between your hands to blend. Label.

To use your hair mask, apply a few drops to your scalp, massaging in small circular motions with your fingertips. Then, using a wide-tooth comb, gently comb from your roots to your ends, saturating your hair and applying more oil if needed, depending on the length and porosity of your hair. Cover with a shower cap and an old towel. Allow the mask to stay on your hair for 30 minutes before rinsing or shampooing it out. Style as usual.

HOT HERBAL BUNDLES

Applying heat to achy muscles improves circulation to the area of soreness and helps alleviate pain and inflammation. In traditional Thai healing, aromatic bundles are first steamed and then applied to the skin while hot to help ease muscles, energize internal organs, and relax the mind. The bundles often include tropical plants such as kaffir lime and lemongrass; however, many of those ingredients can only be found at Asian grocers. So, I also like creating healing bundles with aromatic plants, such as spearmint and basil, that I can grow in my arid climate or purchase in abundance at my Mexican grocer.

I have found that fresh herbs work best and are far more aromatic than dried; however, don't let that keep you from making a bundle. I have yet to go to Thailand to receive this special treatment, but making my own herbal bundles at home is soothing to use on myself and I love giving them as gifts.

Makes 1 bundle

To make 1 bundle, choose any combination of these plants, gathering enough plant material to make roughly the size of a tennis ball, about 1 cup. Plants should be chopped in ½ inch pieces.

Basil	Gingerroot	Rose petals
Calendula	Jasmine flower	Rosemary
Chamomile	Kaffir lime leaves	Spearmint
Culinary sage	Lavender flower	Turmeric root
Eucalyptus	Lemon peel	
Galangal	Orange blossoms	

(continued)

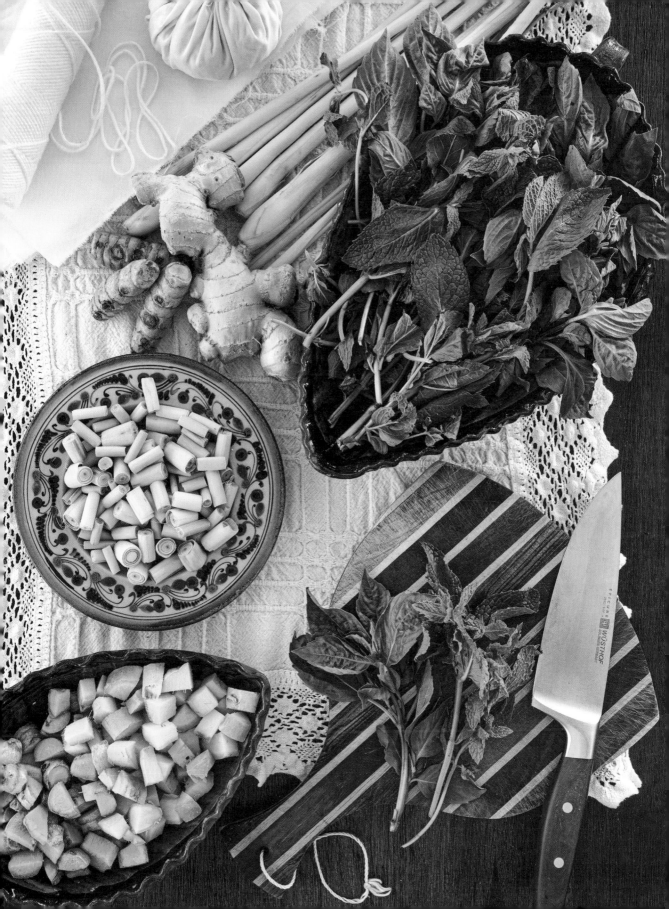

About 1 cup herbs and plants of choice (see page 184)
12-by-12-inch square of cheesecloth or muslin
Electric steamer or bamboo steamer

Put your herb selections into a large mixing bowl and mix well using your hands. Take the mixture and place it in the center of the cloth, making a firm bundle. Secure the bundle with a rubber band or string to create a handle. Be sure it is secured tightly so that it won't become loose when in use. Place the bundle in the steamer, and steam for about 30 minutes.

For application, first check the heat of the bundle on your inner forearm. Once the temperature is to your liking, apply with pressure on areas that are tense and/or painful for up to 15 minutes. You can also lightly dip your steamed bundle in olive oil or coconut oil before application for moisturizing benefits. Store your bundle in the refrigerator in a bag or jar, as it can be used several times before making a new one.

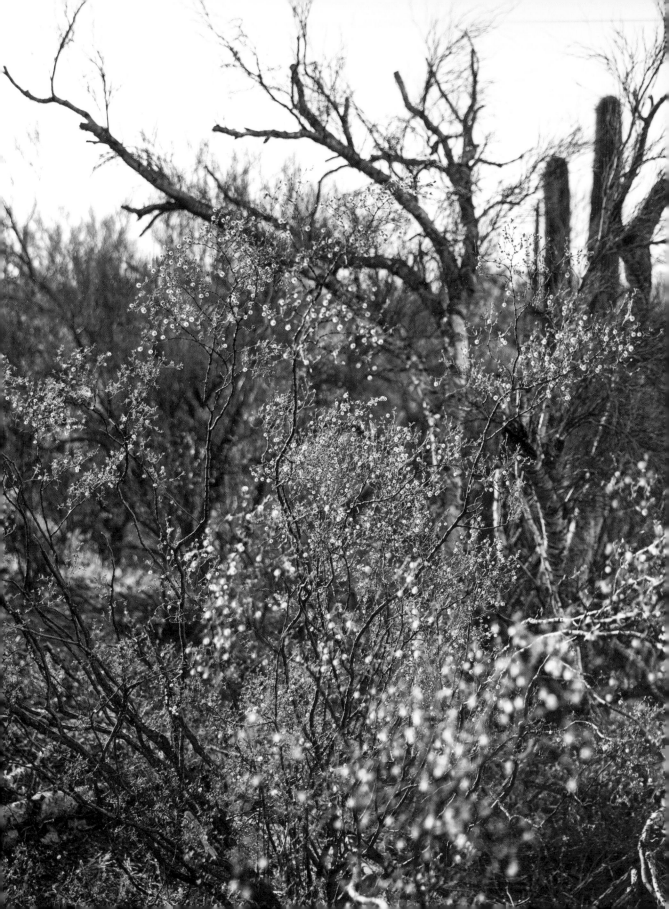

SPIRITUAL WORK WITH FIRE

FIRE HANDS

I've always said that my hands are my greatest tools and using them as a healing tool is no different. Learning to use your hands to cultivate Fire energy is beneficial for self-healing and to transmit healing energy unto others. I first learned this technique by taking Qigong classes long ago, and although it took time, I learned how to create a warm energy between my palms.

I use this technique for my own healing by placing my palms on an area that feels stagnant or sore. I also use this technique as an exercise to play with energy. This ancient modality has been used in Traditional Chinese Medicine for thousands of years for emotional, physical, and spiritual blockages. However, working with Universal Life Force Energy is also used by many other cultures around the world, and it goes by several different names. And for that reason, I simply like to call this technique Fire Hands.

Place your hands in front of your chest as if you were holding a large bowl. You are in a receiving position. Notice your breath and focus on your hands for a few moments, closing your eyes if needed. Next, imagine heat radiating from your palms. Keeping your hands in their curved position, start bringing them together, as in your mind's eye you imagine that you are holding a warm ball of light between your palms. You can move your hands to cradle and handle the ball, taking notice of any feelings of heat. If you move your hands apart and bring them close again, can you feel a tingling sensation? Continue playing with this ball of heat, and when your hands feel warm, you are ready. Place them on the area of your body that you wish to address. Rest them gently on the area and trust your intuition when it's time to remove them.

LETTING GO RITUAL

Since time immemorial, Indigenous people have used smoke as a vessel to carry prayers and thoughts to Creator with the burning of sacred plants such as tobacco, sweetgrass, or Dakota sage. It's moving to watch a bundle of dried plants transform into smoke right before your eyes and it's heartwarming to know the smoke is carrying our thoughts with it. I believe smoke is a powerful messenger; however, it is the flame that ignites the plant, setting into motion transformation for change. So, in the next ritual, the focus is on the flame versus the smoke. Once your paper is ignited by the flame, transformation begins instantly, helping you shift your consciousness and support your being in whatever it is that needs to be released.

On a piece of paper, write down what it is you wish to release. Write as little or as much as your heart feels. When you're done, fold the paper mindfully with the intention of wanting to release the problems, thoughts, or things from your life that you wrote down.

Place a heatproof vessel such as a terracotta pot or cast-iron pan in a safe area and put your folded paper in the bottom of the vessel. Preferably using matches, light your paper. As the fire consumes your paper, visualize all the negativity you wished to be released burn with the flames.

Once the paper has finished burning, allow the vessel and ashes to cool down. Use this opportunity to discard what no longer serves you by scattering the cooled ashes away from you and your space.

SUN-DRYING CLOTHES

This isn't *exactly* spiritual work, but for me, it is work that makes my spirit happy. I absolutely love the way my clothes smell when I hang them out to dry in the sun and find the process quite peaceful. My whites are brighter, it's better for the environment, and this little chore gets me outside for a dose of vitamin D. If you have never put your clothes out to line dry, or haven't done so since you were a child, get some clothesline and laundry pins or a find a drying rack and start harnessing the sun!

A little tip: if you do not want your clothes to feel stiff, add half a cup of white vinegar to your rinse cycle to help dissolve all your detergent. The vinegar scent will disappear as your clothes dry.

Ventosas: Fire Cupping

In recent years, cupping therapy has reemerged with many professional athletes proudly displaying their cupping marks like battle scars after sessions with their acupuncturists, massage therapists, or physical therapists. However, cupping has been practiced all over the world, with traditional healers first using animal horns, bamboo, or clay vessels on their patients instead of rubber, glass, and silicone. There are different types of cupping, sometimes referred to as wet, dry, and fire. In dry and wet cupping, cups are applied to a person's body to gently suction the muscles thus helping release the layer of fascia. In Traditional Chinese Medicine, they are also used to bring vital life force energy to areas of the body where the cups were placed. This is also found in Traditional Mayan Medicine, where the practice of fire cupping is called *ventosas*.

Ventosas help remove "wind" from the body by improving blood stagnation and helping to center your spirit. Done by a trained practitioner, a flame is rapidly placed inside the cup, acting as a heat vacuum, and then taken out immediately, followed by glass being placed on the person's body. The result is a warm, gentle heat that is relaxing to the muscles and beneficial for nervous tension.

Although there are several instances where fire cupping should not be performed, it is a relatively safe practice used since ancient times, with many licensed acupuncturists and trained Traditional Maya practitioners now including it as part of their holistic toolkit to nurture the spirit.

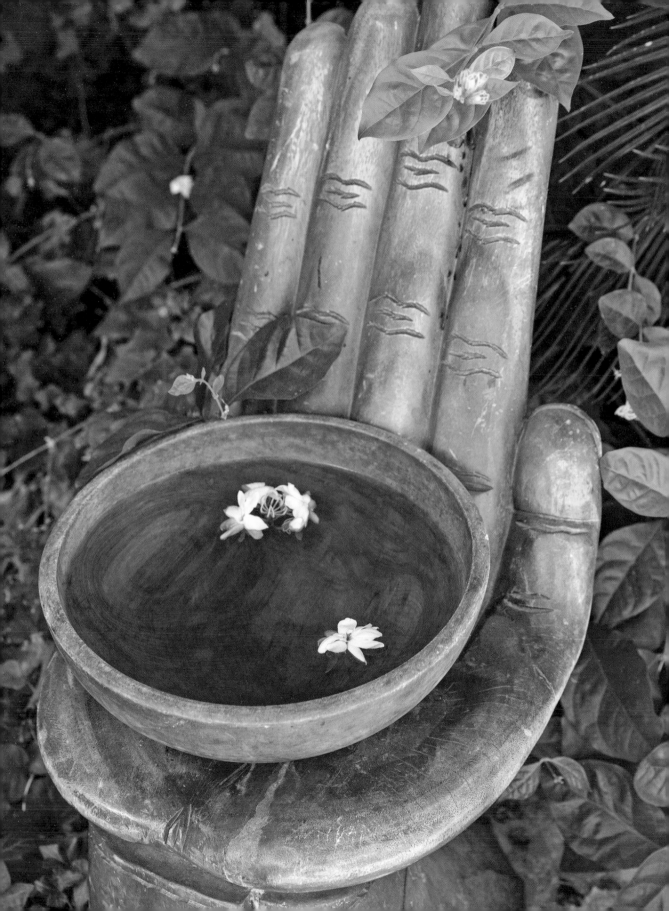

MANZANILLA SUN WASH

Chamomile, known as *manzanilla* in Spanish, is an important plant that is deeply woven into many traditional medicine–ways all over the world. In ancient Egypt, chamomile was held in high regard, with the yellow center of the flower symbolizing the sun god Ra. Many cultures associate chamomile with energy and action, much like the personality of Fire. In my own culture, I was taught that this tiny flower was like the sun itself, bringing joy and relieving anxiety to those who drank it as a tea. One very special way I also like to use manzanilla is to cleanse my body. Not as a bath, but as an herbal infusion poured over my body to banish negativity and bring in more joy. This type of spiritual cleansing is found throughout the Caribbean and Central and South America, using flowers and herbs native to each area. When I take part in the ritual, it feels like a blessing of flowers, reminding me that the sun will rise again the next day.

Makes 1 wash

Large handful of dried or fresh chamomile

Add the chamomile to a medium pot of water. Bring the water to a boil, turn off the heat, cover it with a lid, and infuse the chamomile for 10 minutes. Remove the lid and allow the water to cool completely to room temperature. Strain the herbs, pouring the chamomile water into a safe container such as a plastic bin or stainless steel bowl.

Step into your shower or bathtub and pour the herbal wash over your head while standing in your tub. Allow the chamomile to clear away any negative energy you may be feeling and take in its positive scent like rays of sunshine.

CREATIVE FIRE STARTER

As a holistic aromatherapist, I could say that every essential oil has its own unique personality traits just as people do. One of my personality traits is that I am a fairly creative person. However, usually after a major life change or shift, even I sometimes find myself in a creative funk.

I was trained and believe that specific essential oils fall into certain groups such as calming oils, invigorating oils, and so on based on their aromatic profile and chemical constituents. For example, many people can agree that lavender is relaxing and helps calm the mind. So, when I need to spark my creative fire, I turn to oils that are known to help increase creativity. I prefer to use these oils in an aromatherapy diffuser, so their aromatics can permeate the air around me while I am working and thinking. I also find it's best to choose them intuitively by selecting scents that speak to me at that moment. So, when choosing essential oils to spark your creative fire, close your eyes and select scents that speak to you immediately.

Essential Oils for Creativity

Bergamot	Lemon	Peppermint
Bois de rose	Geranium	Spearmint
Clary sage	Jasmine	Rosemary
Cypress	Juniper	Tangerine
Eucalyptus	Neroli	

There are different types of essential oil diffusers. After choosing a diffuser that is right for you, select one essential oil or a blend of essential oils from the above list and add to your diffuser following the manufacturer's directions. Place your diffuser in a spot where you frequent most and activate your creative fire with one of the affirmations. Run your diffuser as needed.

Creative Fire Affirmations

Divine inspiration surrounds me.

I attract brilliant ideas.

Today, I am filled with infinite creativity.

I take positive action to get things done.

CANDLES IN PRAYER WORK

I often say, "I will light a candle for you" or ask, "What is the person's name you're speaking of?" when I am listening to someone who is sharing a personal dilemma or the news of a loved one who has just passed away. I've always found great power by praying with candles such as lighting votives at various religious shrines or even blowing out candles on my birthday cake. I do not believe candles need to be lit for our prayers to be heard; however, I do believe it's a powerful visual reminder of our intention.

Any candle that is lit with positive intentions holds wisdom within its flame, helping us to go deeper within ourselves when we gaze upon its light. It's as if the candle's light helps reduce the darkness in our minds, and that is why I love candle work so much. They deepen my prayer work.

Choose a candle that speaks to your spirit in color, shape, and scent. My favorite candles for prayer work are simple seven-day white votives in clear glass.

If you like, you can write the person's name on the glass votive with a marker to personalize your prayer or write your intention down on a small piece of paper and tuck it under the base of the candle. Take a deep breath, and as you light your candle, focus your mind on the person or situation you are praying for, stating your intention as you gaze upon its flame. In this moment, connect to your Higher Self, God, Creator, Allah, the Universe, angels, or whatever source from which you draw your spiritual strength, and ask for guidance. And remember, prayers can also be in the form of gratitude. You can always light a candle to simply say "thank you" when you are feeling deep gratitude.

Never leave your candle burning unattended. And each time you relight your candle, state your prayer once again to reignite your intention.

Sample Prayers

May this candle illuminate my path in the midst of my difficulties and decisions.

Creator, please bestow upon me the light of understanding.

I feel gratitude. Thank you.

I pray for peace, harmony, and love among all people.

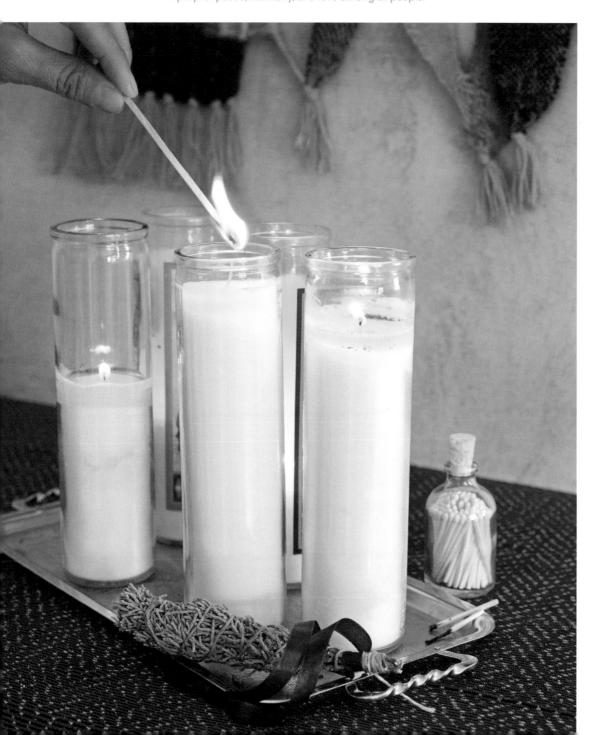

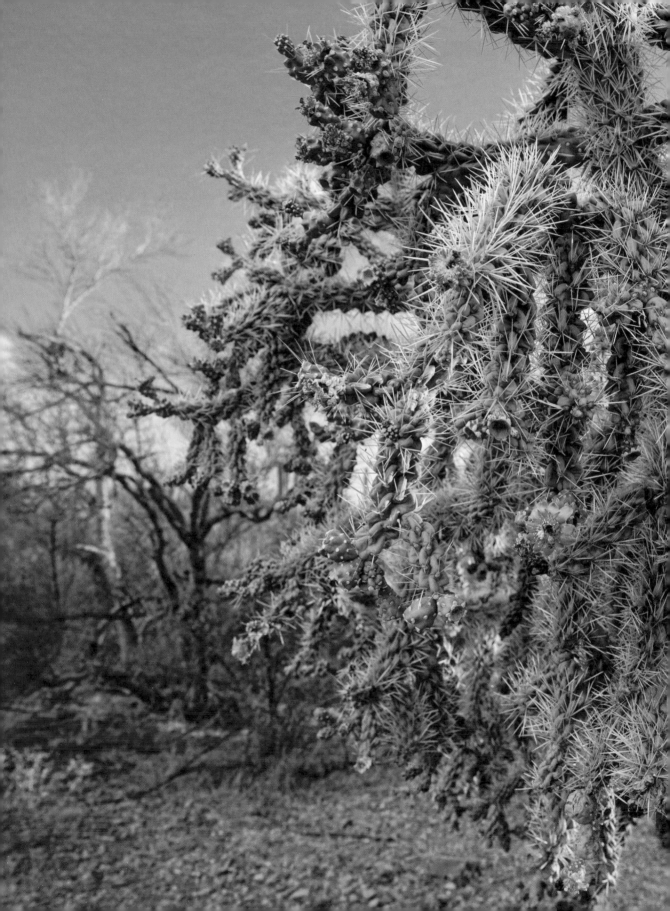

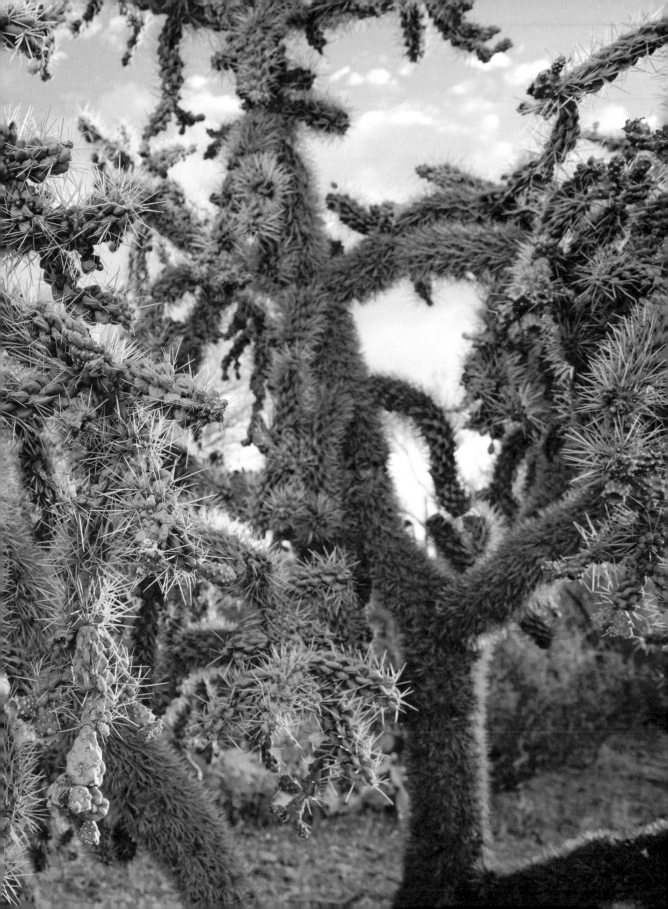

Acknowledgments

First, I would like to thank my husband, Jason, for his endless support in the creation of this book and in life. You truly are my Divine Complement. Words cannot express the gratitude I feel walking alongside a partner who encourages me to be my authentic Self.

A special thank you to my daughter, Paloma, for making me a mother. Breastfeeding you was my first real act of becoming an indigenous foods activist. Thank you for always trying new foods, accompanying me to gatherings, and taking interest in our traditional ways. I pray your heart remains open and you continue learning the wisdom of your ancestors.

Tender love goes out to my twin siblings, Andrea and Diego. Our adventurous childhood gave birth to many of my stories, and I am so grateful I have those memories to reflect on. As the three of us heal from generations of trauma, I am proud of you both for consciously breaking patterns so that we can reclaim and reaffirm who we are for our own children.

I am forever grateful to my comadritas and extended family for supporting my work and vision. Thank you for encouraging my goals, for being recipe testers, photographers, graphic designers, babysitters, builders, genealogists, stylists, models, and most of all, for being a powerful network of advocates that lift me up when needed. You have held my hand through some of my darkest hours, and I consider you all my soulmates. I especially want to thank my Auntie Sara Trujillo for seeing me and my Auntie Mona Polacca, who entered my life during a time when I deeply needed roots.

A special thank you to all my plant teachers, past and present, especially the Indigenous grandmothers of the Southwest who welcomed me into their hearts and kitchens.

I wish to also thank my spiritual teachers, past and present, who have had faith in my work by sharing their teachings with me in circle, especially one of my maestras, friend and curandera Patricia Federico.

ACKNOWLEDGMENTS

I wish to acknowledge my clients, students, and online community for allowing me to shine my light with you in sessions, in workshops, and through social media. I do not exist without you, just as the night does not exist without the day. You all helped me find my voice, and for that, I am deeply grateful.

Nicky Jaan, tashador mikonam vaseyeh honaret va doosteet. / Nicky dear, I thank you for your talents and friendship. What an amazing year it has been putting this creative piece of work together with you! Thank you for seeing ME through your camera's lens.

Lastly, with honor and respect, I give thanks to my ancestors, whose guidance and energy were felt as I worked on this project, always bringing my awareness to a specific subject or memory when I needed. Especially the energy of my dad, Eloy Ruiz, who became an ancestor while I was working on the Air chapter. He shared so many stories of his life with me over the years, and I am grateful that I listened to him as I now know myself even better. To end, I give the highest thanks to Creator for shaping me into my being and providing me with all that I need to live. Tlazocamati!

Felicia Cocotzin Ruiz

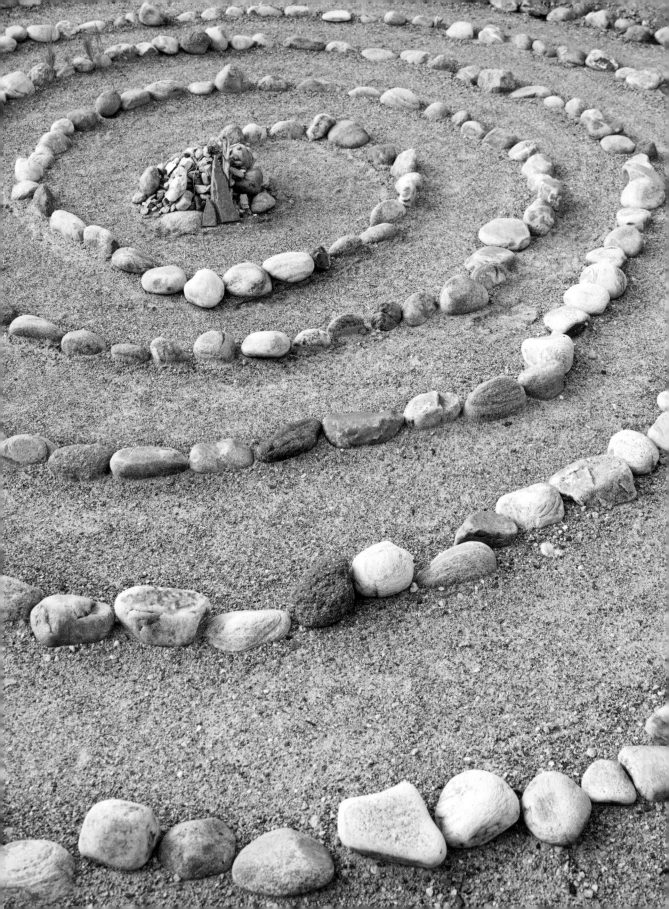

Learn more about indigenous foods and holistic wellness on kitchencurandera.com. In addition, these are websites I frequently visit for information, products, and inspiration.

Aromatherapy

Aromatics.com

LivingLibations.com

PhibeeAromatics.com

SacredWoodEssence.com

Ayurveda

Ayurveda.com

Chopra.com

IAmSaharaRose.com

Curanderismo

Curanderismo.org

Curanderismo.unm.edu

Crystals

ArizonaLapidary.com

CrystalsMtShasta.com

Education

Naha.org

Natifs.org

NewMexico.org

UnitedPlantSavers.org

Herbs

HerbsOfMexico.com

MountainRoseHerbs.com

ScarletSage.com

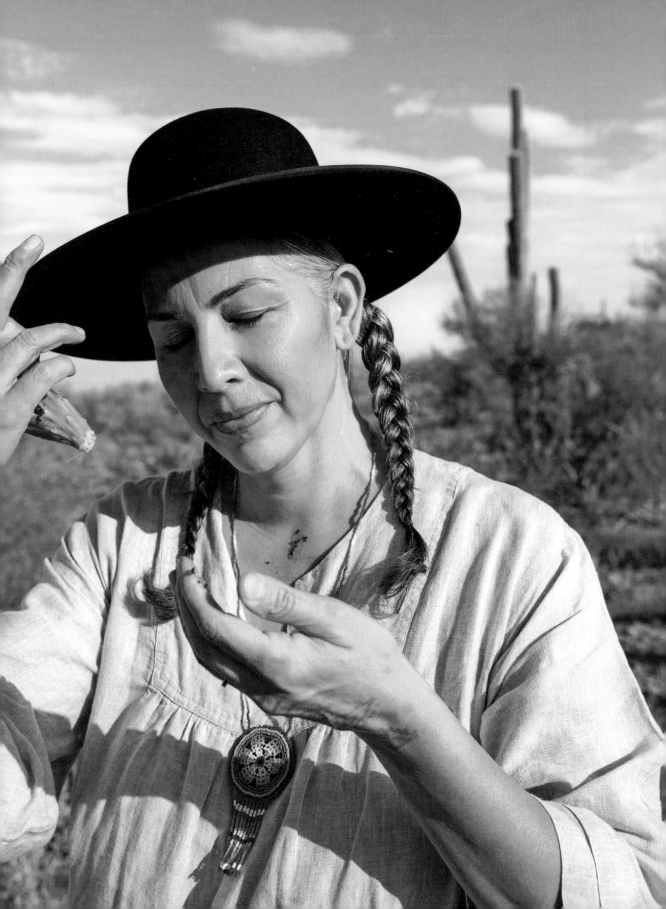

Felicia Cocotzin Ruiz is a traditional healer, storyteller, and indigenous foods activist. As a child, she was deeply influenced by her great-grandmother, who was well-known in her community as a curandera, working with traditional herbs, catching babies, and using her hands to heal. Also called by the healing medicine, Felicia honored her own spirit and began studying massage therapy, energy work, aromatherapy, Indigenous herbalism, whole food cooking, and other holistic modalities, earning the title of Curandera in ceremony in 2018. Felicia lives with her husband in the Sonoran Desert where she works with the sun, the moon, and the elements, offering medicine workshops and one-on-one healing sessions for her community.

Roost Books
An imprint of Shambhala Publications, Inc.
2129 13th Street
Boulder, Colorado 80302
roostbooks.com

The information presented here is thorough and accurate to the best of our knowledge, but it is essential that you always practice caution and use your best judgment when consuming herbs and herbal supplements. Please do not attempt self-treatment of a medical problem without consulting a qualified health practitioner. Shambhala Publications and the author disclaim any and all liability in connection to the consumption of herbs and herbal supplements and the use of the instructions and practices in this book.

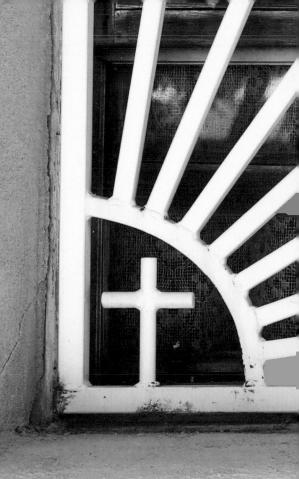

Cover art: Nicky Hedayatzadeh
Design: Kara Plikaitis

9 8 7 6 5 4 3 2

Printed in China

♾This edition is printed on acid-free paper that meets the American National Standards Institute Z39.48 Standard.
♻Shambhala makes every effort to print on postconsumer recycled paper. For more information please visit www.shambhala.com.
Roost Books is distributed worldwide by Penguin Random House, Inc., and its subsidiaries.

Library of Congress Cataloging-in-Publication Data
Names: Ruiz, Felicia Cocotzin, author.

Title: Earth medicines: ancestral wisdom, healing recipes, and wellness rituals from a curandera / Felicia Cocotzin Ruiz ; photographs by Nicky Hedayatzadeh.

Description: First edition. | Boulder, Colorado : Roost Books, [2021] | Includes bibliographical references and index.

Identifiers: LCCN 2020038211 | ISBN 9781611808438 (trade paperback)

Subjects: LCSH: Alternative medicine. | Mind and body.

Classification: LCC R733 .R85 2021 | DDC 610—dc23

LC record available at http://lccn.loc.gov/2020038211